Environmental Health Criteria 2

POLYCHLORINATED BIPHENYLS AND TERPHENYLS

Published under the joint sponsorship of the United Nations Environment Programme and the World Health Organization

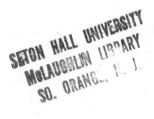

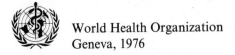

World Health Organization
Geneva, 1976

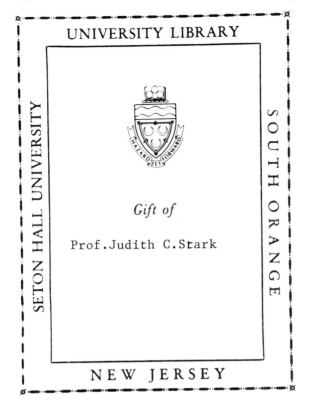
ISBN 92 4 154062 1

PRINTED IN UNITED KINGDOM

CONTENTS

NOTE TO READERS OF THE CRITERIA DOCUMENTS

While every effort has been made to present information in the criteria documents as accurately as possible without unduly delaying their publication, mistakes might have occurred and are likely to occur in the future. In the interest of all users of the environmental health criteria documents, readers are kindly requested to communicate any errors found to the Division of Environmental Health, World Health Organization, Geneva, Switzerland, in order that they may be included in corrigenda which will appear in subsequent volumes.

In addition, experts in any particular field dealt with in the criteria documents are kindly requested to make available to the WHO Secretariat any important published information that may have inadvertently been omitted and which may change the evaluation of health risks from exposure to the environmental agent under examination, so that information may be considered in the event of updating and re-evaluating the conclusions contained in the criteria documents.

WHO TASK GROUP ON ENVIRONMENTAL HEALTH CRITERIA FOR POLYCHLORINATED BIPHENYLS AND TERPHENYLS

Copenhagen, 20–24 October 1975

Participants

Members

Dr V. Beneš, Department of Toxicology, Institute of Hygiene and Epidemiology, Prague, Czechoslovakia (*Vice-Chairman*)

Dr H. L. Falk, National Institute for Environment Health Services, Research Triangle Park, NC, USA

Mr L. Gordts, Institute of Hygiene and Epidemiology, Brussels, Belgium

Dr D. L. Grant, Pesticides Section, Toxicology Evaluation Division, Bureau of Chemical Safety, Department of Health and Welfare, Ottawa, Ontario, Canada (*Rapporteur*)

Mr A. V. Holden, Department of Agriculture and Fisheries for Scotland, Freshwater Fisheries Laboratory, Faskally, Pitlochry, Perthshire, Scotland

Dr S. Jensen, Naturvardsverkets Specialanalytiska Laboratorium, Wallenberg-laboratoriet, Lilla Frescati, Stockholm, Sweden

Dr Renate Kimbrough, Center for Disease Control, Toxicology Branch, Atlanta, GA, USA

Professor H. Kuratsune, Department of Public Health, Faculty of Medicine, Kyushu University, Fukuoka, Japan

Dr E. Schulte, Institut für Lebensmittelchemie der Westfälischen Wilhelms-Universität, Münster/Westf., Federal Republic of Germany

Dr J. G. Vos, Laboratory for Pathology, National Institute for Public Health, Bilthoven, Netherlands (*Chairman*)

Observer

Dr D. Axelrod, Division of Laboratories and Research, New York State Department of Health, Albany, NY, USA

Unable to attend
   [a] Dr M. V. Kryžanovskaja, All-Union Institute for Research on Hygiene and Toxicology of Pesticides, Polymers, and Plastics, Kiev, USSR.

Representatives of other organizations:

International Federation of Pharmaceutical Manufacturers Associations
Professor P. Fabiani, Laboratoire du Chimie et de Toxicologie de l'Hôtel Dieu, Paris, France

Permanent Commission and International Association on Occupational Health
Dr Aa. Grut, State Labour Inspection Service, Hellerup, Denmark

Secretariat:

Dr J. C. Gage, 21 Lambolle Road, London, England (*Temporary Adviser*)

Dr M. J. Suess, Environmental Pollution Control, WHO Regional Office for Europe, Copenhagen, Denmark

Dr A. H. Wahba, Health Laboratory Services, WHO Regional Office for Europe, Copenhagen, Denmark

Dr G. Vettorazzi, Food Additives Unit, Division of Environmental Health, World Health Organization, Geneva (*Secretary*)

Dr D. C. Villeneuve,[a] Laboratory of Toxicology, National Institute of Public Health, Bilthoven, Netherlands (*Temporary Adviser*)

---

[a] On sabbatical leave from: Biochemical Toxicology Unit, Environmental Toxicology Division, Environmental Health Centre, Department of Health and Welfare, Ottawa, Ontario, Canada.

ENVIRONMENTAL HEALTH CRITERIA FOR POLYCHLORINATED BIPHENYLS AND TERPHENYLS

A WHO Task Group on Environmental Health Criteria for Polychlorinated Biphenyls (PCBs) and Terphenyls (PCTs) met in Copenhagen from 20-24 October 1975. Dr F. A. Bauhofer, Director of Health Services of the WHO Regional Office for Europe opened the meeting on behalf of the Director-General and the Director of the Regional Office for Europe. The Task Group reviewed and amended the second draft criteria document and made an evaluation of the health risks from exposure to these compounds.

The preparation of the first draft criteria document was based on national reviews of health effects research on polychlorinated biphenyls, received from the national focal points collaborating in the WHO Environmental Health Criteria Programme in Canada, the Federal Republic of Germany, Finland, France, Japan, the Netherlands, New Zealand, Sweden, the United Kingdom, and the USA. Dr J. C. Gage, London, England, prepared the first draft as well as the second draft criteria document which took into account the comments received from the national focal points in Canada, Czechoslovakia, the Federal Republic of Germany, France, Japan, New Zealand, Sweden, the United Kingdom, the USA, and the USSR; from the United Nations Industrial Development Organization (UNIDO), Vienna, the Food and Agriculture Organization of the United Nations (FAO) Rome, and from the United Nations Educational, Scientific and Cultural Organization (UNESCO) Paris; the Organization for Economic Co-operation and Development, Paris, and the Health Protection Directorate of the Commission of the European Communities, Luxembourg.

Comments were also received at the request of the Secretariat, from Dr K. Kojima, Japan, Dr D. S. May, United Kingdom, and Dr V. Zitko, Canada.

The collaboration of these national institutions, international organizations and individual experts is gratefully acknowledged. Without their assistance the document could not have been completed.

This document is based primarily on original publications listed in the reference section. In addition, some recent publications reviewing the environmental and health aspects of polychlorinated biphenyls were also used. These include reviews by the Commission of the European Communities (1974), the US Department of Health, Education and

Welfare (1972), the International Agency for Research on Cancer (1974), the International Council for the Exploration of the Sea (1974), Jensen (1974), Kimbrough (1974), the National Swedish Environment Protection Board (1973), the Panel on Hazardous Trace Substances (1972), the USDA/USDC/EPA/FDA/USDA (1972), and a WHO working group (1973).

Details about the WHO Environmental Health Criteria Programme including the definition of some terms frequently used in the document may be found in the general introduction to the Environmental Health Criteria Programme published together with the Environmental Health Criteria Document on mercury (Environmental Health Criteria 1, Geneva World Health Organization, 1976).

1. SUMMARY AND RECOMMENDATIONS FOR FURTHER RESEARCH

1.1 Introductory Note

The commercial production of the polychlorinated biphenyls (PCBs) began in 1930, and during the 1930s cases of poisoning were reported among men engaged in their manufacture. The nature of this occupational disease was characterized by a skin affliction with acneiform eruptions; occasionally the liver was involved, in some cases with fatal consequences. Subsequent safety precautions appear largely to have prevented further outbreaks of this disease in connection with the manufacture of PCBs, but from 1953 onwards, cases have been reported in Japanese factories manufacturing condensers.

The distribution of PCBs in the environment was not recognized until Jensen started an investigation in 1964 to ascertain the origins of unknown peaks observed during the gas–liquid chromatographic separation of organochlorine pesticides from wild-life samples. In 1966, he and his colleagues succeeded in attributing these to the presence of PCBs. Since that time, investigations in many parts of the world have revealed the widespread distribution of PCBs in environmental samples.

The serious outbreaks of poisoning in man and in domestic animals from the ingestion of food accidentally contaminated with PCBs have stimulated investigations into the toxic effects of PCBs on animals and on nutritional food chains. This has resulted in limitation of the commercial exploitation of PCBs and polychlorinated terphenyls (PCTs), and in regulations to limit the residues in human and animal food.

The environmental impact of the PCBs and PCTs has been the subject of several reviews, and has been discussed at a number of regional and international meetings. The relevant publications are mentioned in the previous section.

1.2 Summary

1.2.1 Composition and analytical problems

The commercial production of PCBs and PCTs by the direct chlorination of biphenyl and terphenyl leads to a mixture of components with a range of chlorine contents, the mean percentage chlorine in the product being controlled to give the required technical properties. Most of these components have been separated by gas–liquid chromatography, and the PCBs in the mixtures have been characterized after synthesis of the

11

components by unequivocal routes. Techniques are available to analyse environmental samples for PCBs and PCTs, and experience has shown that interlaboratory collaborative studies are necessary to establish competence to determine residues below the 1 mg/kg level.

The commercial PCB mixtures contain various quantities of impurities, among which chlorinated dibenzofurans and chlorinated naphthalenes have been identified.

1.2.2   Sources and pathways in the environment

The estimated cumulative world production of PCBs since 1930 is of the order of 1 million tonnes. Of this, more than one-half has entered dumps and landfills, where it is likely to be stable and released only very slowly. Much of the remainder has entered the environment by the disposal of industrial fluids into rivers and coastal waters, by leakage from nonenclosed systems, or by volatilization into the atmosphere from incineration of PCB-containing material at dumps. The ultimate reservoirs of PCBs and PCTs that enter the environment are mainly sediments of rivers and coastal waters. PCBs and PCTs are stable in the environment, but a small proportion is transformed by biological action and possibly by photolysis.

1.2.3   Concentration in the environment

Measured concentrations of PCBs in air range from 50 ng/m^3 to less than 1 ng/m^3. Nonpolluted fresh waters should contain less than 0.5 ng of PCBs per litre compared with 50 ng per litre in moderately polluted rivers and estuaries, and 500 ng per litre in highly polluted rivers. The concentration in living organisms depends upon the extent of local pollution, the amount of fat in the tissues, and the trophic stage of the organism in food chains. Highest tissue levels were found in marine ecosystems with very high values in top predators from polluted areas, though most of the fish caught for human consumption contains PCBs at levels of less than 0.1 mg/kg in muscle tissue. There is no information available on the environmental distribution of PCTs.

1.2.4   Metabolism

PCBs are well absorbed by mammals through the gastrointestinal tract, lungs, and skin. They are stored mainly in adipose tissue and there is some placental transfer. Excretion in mammals is mainly through faeces, where the PCBs appear as phenolic metabolites; they appear unchanged in human milk. In birds, there is a considerable excretion in eggs. The rate of excretion in faeces is dependent on the rate of metabolism and this is much influenced by the number and orientation of the chlorine substituents. As environmental PCBs pass up biological food chains, there is a progressive loss of the lower chlorinated components owing to selective biotransformation, and only traces of PCBs containing less than five chlorine atoms per molecule are found in human fat.

The smaller amount of information available concerning the PCTs indicates that they also are absorbed from the gastrointestinal tract and undergo selective biotransformation, but that the concentration in fat in relation to that in other tissues appears to be less than is observed with the PCBs.

1.2.5 The extent of human exposure

Surveys on human adipose tissue in several countries have shown that most samples contain levels of PCBs in the region of 1 mg/kg or less, although higher values have been reported from some countries. Much higher values, up to 700 mg/kg, have been found in fat from men occupationally exposed. Several national surveys give PCB concentrations in the blood in the region of 0.3 μg/100 ml but levels approaching 200 μg/100 ml have been measured in men occupationally exposed, and these may be associated with skin lesions. Most surveys on human milk have shown PCB concentrations in the region of 0.02 mg/litre, although concentrations up to 0.1 mg/litre have been recorded. Results from the very few investigations on PCT concentrations in fat and blood suggest that these may be equal to those of PCBs.

An estimate of the total daily intake of PCBs in air, water, and diet by individuals not occupationally exposed indicates that this falls within the range of 5–100 μg, which may be supplemented by unknown amounts from nondietary sources. This estimate has some support from measurements of concentrations in human milk.

1.2.6 Experimental studies on the effects of PCBs and PCTs

Most of the studies on the toxicity of PCBs have been performed with the commercial mixtures. The PCBs are of low acute toxicity but the effects are cumulative with prolonged administration; in mammals, liver enlargement is observed that may progress to liver damage. Non-metastasizing neoplastic liver nodules have been produced in rats and mice, some of which were classified as hepatocellular carcinomas on the basis of histological criteria in one study in rats and one study in mice.

The monkey is much more sensitive to PCBs than the rat, showing effects similar to those seen in human Yusho patients (See section 8, p 65) with a similar order of exposure. Low dose effects on fertility have been seen in both the monkey and the mink, a species that is also relatively sensitive to PCBs.

Other effects of PCBs include porphyria, immunosuppression, and interference with steroid metabolism; some of these may be attributable to the increase in microsomal enzyme activity associated with liver enlargement. Some of the toxic effects can be attributed to impurities in the commercial products.

The toxicity of PCBs to fish is not high by comparison with that of some pesticides, but some aquatic invertebrates are more sensitive. There is little information on the toxicity of the PCTs.

1.2.7   Clinical studies of the effects of PCBs in man

Information on the effects of PCBs in man has been obtained from a large-scale incident in Japan (Yusho), in which over 1000 individuals showed signs of poisoning from the ingestion of rice oil contaminated with PCBs from a heat exchanger liquid. The most striking effects were hypersecretion in the eyes, pigmentation and acneiform eruptions of the skin, and disturbances of the respiratory system. Babies born to Yusho mothers were of less than normal size and initially showed skin pigmentation. Over a six-year period, the effects on the skin diminished very gradually, but the nonspecific symptoms tended to become somewhat more prominent. The smallest dose of PCBs calculated to produce an effect was approximately 0.5 g over about 120 days, but as the rice oil contained chlorinated dibenzofurans at a concentration of 5 mg/kg of rice oil in addition to PCBs at 2000–3000 mg/kg it is not certain that the symptoms were due solely to PCBs.

1.2.8   Dose–effect relationships

Experimental studies on the dose–effect relationship have shown that no effects on growth, and reproduction are seen in rats receiving PCB levels of 1 mg/kg body weight per day; there may be liver enlargement and a reversible induction of microsome enzyme activity at a level of 1 mg/kg/day but not at 0.1 mg/kg/day. Effects on reproduction are seen in the monkey with PCB levels of about 0.12 mg/kg/day. Symptoms were reported in some Yusho patients ingesting less than 0.1 mg/kg/day.

1.3 Recommendations for Further Research

1.3.1 Analytical methods

Collaborative intercalibration studies on the determination of PCBs, PCTs, and chlorinated dibenzofurans should be established between all laboratories engaged in determining these compounds in environmental samples, and adequate standards should be made available for individual chlorinated biphenyls and dibenzofurans.

Improved analytical techniques, including those involving capillary gas–liquid chromatography and mass spectroscopy, should be developed for the determination of PCBs, PCTs, polybrominated biphenyls, polychlorinated dibenzofurans, and naphthalenes, and their metabolites and degradation products.

1.3.2 Environmental pollution

The content of chlorinated dibenzofurans should be studied in a range of commercial PCB mixtures, and in used PCBs from existing or newly designed heat exchangers, capacitors, and hydraulic transmissions. The possibility of the formation of chlorinated dibenzofurans from PCBs in cooking oils before and after use and in other foods during storage or heating requires investigation.

The current production, use patterns, and methods of disposal of PCBs should be carefully examined to gain information on the impact of PCBs on the environment at the present time. The rate of leaching of PCBs from waste dumps and landfills should be studied, and methods of incineration should be investigated to ascertain which of the components survive inefficient combustion, and whether chlorinated dibenzofurans or other compounds are released into the atmosphere.

Information is required on the metabolism and environmental fate of the chlorinated dibenzofurans.

1.3.3 Effects on man

The intake of PCBs and PCTs from all sources by typical populations should be studied, and an attempt should be made to trace the sources of PCBs and PCTs in those items of the diet that make the greatest contribution to the daily intake. Further measurements are required on levels in human body fat, blood, and milk, and an attempt should be made to relate these levels to the daily intake.

Clinical and epidemiological studies are required on individuals exposed to relatively high concentrations of PCBs and PCTs, either occupationally or by virtue of the nature of their diet, and their health status should be correlated with exposure and tissue levels.

1.3.4   Experimental studies

Further toxicological and metabolic studies are required on individual polychlorinated biphenyls, dibenzofurans, naphthalenes, and other impurities occurring in commercial products, on a variety of species including primates, in order to assess the nature of the toxic effects, the dose–response relationship, and the threshold of toxic effects. Such investigations should be extended to include dermal and inhalation exposure.

Carcinogenic and cocarcinogenic studies should be undertaken to identify the components in commercial PCBs responsible for neoplastic effects.

1.3.5   PCB substitutes

More information should be made available on the production and use patterns of PCTs, polybrominated biphenyls, and of other possible substitutes for PCBs, and when appropriate, these products should be subjected to adequate toxicological investigations.

2. PROPERTIES AND ANALYTICAL METHODS

2.1   Chemical Composition

The PCBs form a class of chlorinated hydrocarbons and are manu-factured commercially by the progressive chlorination of biphenyl in the presence of a suitable catalyst. They are known by a variety of trade names: Aroclor (USA), Phenochlor (France), Clophen (Federal Republic of Germany), Kanechlor (Japan), Fenchlor (Italy), and Sovol (USSR). Their value for industrial applications depends upon their chemical inertness, resistance to heat, non-flammability, low vapour pressure (particularly with the higher chlorinated compounds), and high dielectric constant. There are many different trade names for mixtures of PCBs with other compounds.

Individual manufacturers have their own system of identification for their products. In the Aroclor series, a four digit code is used; biphenyls are generally indicated by 12 in the first two positions, while the last two numbers indicate the percentage by weight of chlorine in the mixture; thus Aroclor 1260 is a polychlorinated-biphenyl mixture containing 60% of chlorine. An exception to this generalization is Aroclor 1016 which is a distillation product of Aroclor 1242 containing only 1% of components with five or more chlorine atoms (Burse et al., 1974). With other commercial products the codes may indicate the approximate mean number of chlorine atoms in the components; thus Clophen A60, Phenochlor DP6, and Kanechlor 600 are biphenyls with an average of about six chlorine atoms per molecule (equivalent to 59.0% chlorine by weight).

In the Aroclor series, terphenyls are indicated by 54 in the first two places of the four digit code. In Japan, the PCTs are coded Kanechlor KC-C.

Individual PCBs have been synthesized for use as reference samples in the identification of gas–liquid chromatographic peaks, for toxicological investigations, and for studying their metabolic fate in living organisms, for which purpose they have been prepared labelled with carbon-14 (Hutzinger et al., 1971; Tas & de Vos, 1971; Webb & McCall, 1972; Moron, et al., 1972; Sundström & Wachtmeister, 1973; Jensen & Sundström, 1974).

The chlorination of biphenyl can lead to the replacement of 1–10 hydrogen atoms by chlorine; the conventional numbering of substituent positions is shown in the diagram. It has been calculated that 210 different

biphenyls of different chlorine content are theoretically possible, although Sissons & Welti (1971) have demonstrated that chlorine substituents in the 3,5- and 2,4,6-positions are not obtained by the direct chlorination of biphenyl. The proportions of PCBs with 1–9 chlorine substituents in the Aroclors are shown in Table 1.

There have been several investigations to identify individual PCBs in commercial products. Sissons & Welti (1971) separated the components of the Aroclors by column and gas–liquid chromatography, and characterized many of the peaks by high-resolution mass spectrometry and nuclear magnetic resonance, and by comparison with 40 synthesized

Table 1. Approximate composition of Aroclors

No. of Cl atoms in molecule	% of chlorine weight	Aroclor 1221[a]	1242[b]	1248[b]	1254[b]	1260[b]
0	0	12.7				
1	18.8	47.1	3			
2	31.8	32.3	13	2		
3	41.3		28	18		
4	48.6		30	40	11	
5	54.4		22	36	49	12
6	59.0		4	4	34	38
7	62.8				6	41
8	66.0					8
9	68.8					1

[a] Willis & Addison (1972).
[b] Panel on Hazardous Trace Substances (1972).

Table 2. Polychlorinated biphenyls in Aroclors 1221–1254 (Webb & McCall, 1972)

Retention time[a]	Synthetic chlorobiphenyl	Aroclor 1221	1232	1242	1248	1254
10	Biphenyl	×[b] C[c]	×	×	×	
13	2	× C	×	×	×	
16.9	3	× D[d]				
17	4	× C	×			
17.7				×		
18.5	2,2'	× C	×	× C	×	
21.3		×	×	×		
21.6		×	×	×		
23.5	2,3'	× C	×	×	×	
24	2,4'	× C	×	×	×	
26	2,6,2'		×	× D	×	
29	2,5,2'		×	× C	×	
29.2	2,4,2'	×	×	× C	×	
29.5	4,4'	× C	×	× C	×	
34	2,3,2'		×	× C[e]	×	
38	2,4,3'		×	× C	×	
38.5	2,4,4'		×	× C	×	
38.7	2,5,4'		×	× C	×	
41.5				×	×	
42.5	3,4,2'			× C	×	
43				×	×	
44				×	×	
44.5					×	
48	2,5,2',5'			× C	×	× C
49.5	2,4,2',5'			× C	×	× C
50.5	2,4,2',4'			× D	×	
51.5				×	×	
55	2,3,2',5'			×	×	× C
57				×	×	
59	2,3,6,2',6'			×	×	× D

Retention time[a]	Synthetic chlorobiphenyl	Aroclor 1221	1232	1242	1248	1254
60				×	×	
64				×	×	
69				×	×	
69.5					×	×
70	2,5,3',4'			× C[e]	×	
70.5	2,3,6,2',5'					× C
71	2,4,3',4'			× C[e]	×	
72				×	×	
76	2,3,6,2',4'					× C
82					×	
83	2,3,6,2',3'				×	× C
84					×	
85	2,4,5,2',5'				×	× C
87	2,4,5,2',4'				×	× C
96						×
99	2,4,5,2',3'				×	× C
101					×	×
104					×	×
107	2,3,6,3',4'				×	×
115						×
117					×	×
119						×
125	2,4,5,2',3',6'					× C
126	2,4,5,3',4'				×	× C
135						×
147						×
148	2,4,5,2',4',5'					× C
149						×
152						×
165						×
178						×

[a] Relative to p,p'–DDE at 190°C on 100' × 0.02' SCOT SE 30 column.

[b] × indicates a GLC peak in this Aroclor at this retention time.

[c] C means that the synthetic compound in the second column was confirmed by GLC and IR in this Aroclor. Because of the labour involved, most compounds were only confirmed in one Aroclor. For example, biphenyl is probably present in 1232–1248 as well as 1221.

[d] Only GLC data available.

[e] Something else also present.

18

PCBs. Webb & McCall (1972) identified the gas–liquid chromatographic peaks with those of synthesized compounds by retention times and infrared spectrometry (Table 2). The most exhaustive study is that of Jensen & Sundström (1974). They recognized that conventional gas–liquid chromatography could not separate all the components, so they devised a preliminary fractionation on a charcoal column, which separated the component PCBs according to the number of chlorines in the 2,2′,6 or 6′ positions in the molecule (o-chlorines). They compared the gas–liquid chromatographic peaks with those of 90 synthesized PCBs, and were able to characterize and quantify 60 components of Clophens A50 and A60 (Table 3). Tables 2 and 3 show a considerable overlap between the components of Aroclor 1254 and Clophen A50.

2.2 Purity of Products

Commercial PCBs are not sold on a composition specification, but on their physical properties. Different batches may vary somewhat from the compositions shown in Tables 1–3. Impurities known to be present in commercial PCBs are chlorinated dibenzofurans and chlorinated naphthalenes (Vos et al., 1970; Bowes et al., 1975). Bowes et al. (1975) found chlorinated dibenzofurans at 0.8–2.0 mg/kg in samples of the Aroclor 1248–1260 series, but none in Aroclor 1016, and at levels of 8.4 mg/kg in Clophen A60 and 13.6 mg/kg in Phenoclor DP–6. Roach & Pomerantz (1974) found chlorinated dibenzofurans levels of 1 mg/kg and Nagayama et al. (1976) found 18 mg/kg in different batches of Kanechlor 400, but no chlorinated dibenzodioxins.

2.3 Determination of PCB Residues

Reviews have been published on methods used for the determination of organochlorine compounds including PCBs in environmental samples (Holden, 1973a, Panel on Hazardous Trace Substances, 1972). No two laboratories have identical methods, although all have features in common. The techniques appear to be those previously developed for the determination of organochlorine pesticides with appropriate modifications for the presence of PCBs, and the studies on PCBs sometimes form part of a wider programme for monitoring persistent organochlorine compounds in the environment. The major difficulties in the determination of PCBs are to separate them from interfering organochlorine pesticides, and to derive a single quantitative figure from a variable mixture of components.

Table 3. Percentages of polychlorinated biphenyls in Clophen A50 and A60 and in human fat (Jensen & Sundström, 1974)

No.	Structure[a]	No. of ortho-chlorines	Relative retention time Apiezon L	SF 96	Percentage in Clophen A50	A60	Human tissue
1	2,5–2'5'	2	0.25	0.30	5.0		
2	2,4–2'5'	2	0.26	0.30	1.4		
3	2,3–2'5'	2	0.27	0.33	1.9		1.1
4	(2,–2',3',4')	2	0.30	0.43	1.2		0.66
5	(4–2',3'6')	2	0.32	0.43	2.1		0.56
6	2,5–2',3',6'	3	0.35	0.43	4.4[b]	2.9	1.2
7	2,3–2',3',6'	3	0.38	0.49	2.5[b]	0.28	0.48
8	3,4–2',5'	1	0.41	0.42	3.9		1.5
9		1 or 2	0.42		2.2[c]		2.0[c]
10	2,5–2',3',5'	2	0.45	0.49	2.2	1.1	1.2
11	2,3,6–2',3',6'	4	0.47	0.61	0.50	1.0[d]	
12	2,5–2',4',5'	2	0.48	0.50	7.0[b]	5.6	4.2
13	2,4–2',4',5'	2	0.51	0.51	1.8[b]	—[e]	1.9
14	2,3–2',4',5'	2	0.53	0.57	1.4[b]		
15	2,5–2',3',4'	2	0.53	0.58	5.4	1.4	2.3
16	2,3–2',3',4'	2	0.55	0.66	1.0		
17	3,4–2',3',6'	2	0.56	0.62	7.6[b]	2.9	4.7
18	2,3,5–2',3',6'	3	0.60	0.70	1.2	4.2	1.0
19	2,4,5–2',3',6'	3	0.64	0.73	2.0[b]	6.5[d]	0.13
20	2,5–2',3',5',6'	3	0.65	0.68	1.3	3.3	0.43
21	2,3–2',3',5',6'	3	0.70	0.74	0.5		0.05
22	2,3,4–2',3',6'	3	0.72	0.83	1.8	3.2	0.15
23		1 or 2	0.76		0.6[c]		
24	2,3,6–2',3',5',6'	4	0.77	0.91	0.09	0.96	
25	3,4–2',4',5'	1	0.79	0.74	5.0[b]	1.6	5.4
26	2,3,6–2',3'4',6'	4	0.84	0.95	0.05	0.37	
27	2,3,5–2',4',5'	2	0.85	0.86	0.90	2.9	2.7
28	3,4–2',3',4'	1	0.87	0.86	3.6		1.9
29	2,4,5–2',4',5'	2	0.90	0.86	4.2[b]	12.9[d]	21.5
30	2,3,4–2',3',5'	2	0.94	0.97 }	1.1	1.5	—[e]
31		1 or 2	0.96	0.93 }		—[e]	
32	2,3,4–2',4',5'	2	1.00	1.00	5.1	11.3[d]	14.0
33	2,3,5–2',3',5',6'	3	1.01	1.06	0.04	0.49	0.90
34		4	1.02		0.05[c]		
35		1 or 2	1.04	1.10	1.1[c]	2.0[c]	1.5[c]
36	2,4,5–2',3',5',6'	3	1.08	1.13	0.39	3.3	3.5

2.3.1 Extraction of sample

Air

Particulate fallout from air has been trapped on 200 μm nylon net coated with silicone oil, and the PCBs then extracted with hexane (Södergren, 1972a). Separate determinations of particulate and vapour phase PCBs in air have been made by the passage of a large volume of air through a filter which was followed by an impinger containing hexane (Hasegawa et al., 1972b), or a polyurethane plug (Bidleman & Olney, 1974) or ceramic saddles coated with OV 17 silicone (Harvey & Steinhauer, 1974) to absorb the vapour.

Water

PCBs have been extracted from water by passing a sample through a

Table 3.—continued

Compound		No. of ortho-chlorines	Relative retention time		Percentage in		Human tissue
					Clophen		
No.	Structure[a]		Apiezon L	SF 96	A50	A60	
37	2,3,4–2',3',4'	2	1.11	1.16	1.3	2.0	0.81
38	2,3,6–2',3',4',5'	3	1.13	1.29	0.33	3.7[d]	—[e]
39	2,4,5–2',3',4',6'	3	1.14	1.16	0.17	1.8	2.5
40	2,3,4–2',3',5',6'	3	1.19	1.32	0.27	2.1	1.3
41	2,3,5,6–2',3',5',6'	4	1.23	1.34	0.005	0.07	
42	2,3,4–2',3',4',6'	3	1.28	1.40	0.13	1.3	0.57
43	2,3,4,6–2',3',5',6'	4	1.34	1.44	0.007	0.09	
44	2,4,5–3',4',5'	1	1.41	1.19	0.47	1.0	0.49
45	2,3,6–2',3',4',5',6'	4	1.45	1.59	0.008	0.09	
46	2,3,4,6–2',3',4',6'	4	1.46	1.51	—[e]	0.03	
47	3,4–2',3',4',5'	1	1.55	1.37	0.81	1.5	2.0
48	2,3,5–2',3',4',5'	2	1.59	1.49	0.23	0.90	1.2
49	2,4,5–2',3',4',5'	2	1.71	1.56	0.98	7.6[d]	7.7
50	2,3,4–2',3',4',5'	2	1.88	1.82	0.72	4.1[d]	5.9
51	2,3,4,5–2',3',5',6'	3	1.94	1.99	0.08	0.74	0.77
52		1 or 2	2.02	1.96	0.23[c]	1.0[c]	—[e]
53	2,3,4,5–2',3',4',6'	3	2.07	2.05	0.06	0.44	0.94
54	2,4,5–2',3',4',5',6'	3	2.15	2.04	0.01	0.28	0.46
55	(2,3,5,6–2',3',4',5',6')	4	2.23				—[e]
56	2,3,4–2',3',4',5',6'	3	2.40	2.20	0.01	0.17	0.31
57	2,3,4,6–2',3',4',5',6'	4	2.45	2.56	—[e]	—[e]	—[e]
58	3,4,5–2',3',4',5'	1	2.74	2.41	—[e]	—[e]	
59	2,3,4,5–2',3',4',5'	2	3.18	2.81	0.35	0.67	1.7
60	2,3,4,5,6–2',3',4',5',6'4	4	4.12				0.62
				Total	86.7%	99.4%	100.0%
	p,p'–DDE		0.52	0.58			
	p,p'–DDT		0.71	0.73			
	p,p'–DDT		0.90	0.97			

[a] Tentative structures are given in brackets.

[b] Component found present in Aroclor 1254 by Webb & McCall (1972).

[c] Figures calculated using responses of chlorobiphenyls with similar retention times in the same fraction from the charcoal column.

[d] Component found present in Phenoclor DP6 by Tas & Vos (1971).

[e] Present in trace amounts only.

filter of undecane and Carbowax 400 monostearate supported on Chromosorb W (Ahling & Jensen, 1970) or a porous plug of polyurethane coated with a suitable gas–liquid chromatographic stationary phase (Uthe et al., 1972), or Amberlite XAD–2 resin (Harvey, et al., 1973) followed by elution of the PCBs with a solvent. Anhoff & Josefsson (1975) have described a liquid–liquid extraction into cyclohexane.

Biological samples

Most analysts have used standard methods developed for organochlorine pesticides, in which the PCBs are extracted together with the fat; the sample is ground with anhydrous sodium sulphate and extracted with petroleum ether or hexane. Porter et al. (1970) studied the optimal conditions for this procedure. A dehydrating solvent may be included to facilitate the breakdown of cell structures; ethanol (Norén & Westöö,

21

1968) and acetone (Jensen et al., 1973) have been used. Rote & Murphy (1971) digested the sample with a mixture of acetic and perchloric acids prior to hexane extraction.

2.3.2 Clean-up

Methods for the removal of fat from the extract include solvent partitioning between hexane and acetonitrile or dimethylformamide, or treatment with strong sulfuric acid or ethanolic potassium hydroxide. Gel permeation has also been used (Stalling et al., 1972), and Holden & Marsden (1969) removed fat on dry, partially deactivated alumina columns. Certain pesticides such as dieldrin are destroyed by the sulfuric acid treatment, so this method cannot be used if such pesticides are to be determined together with PCBs (Jensen et al., 1973).

PCBs may be separated from organochlorine pesticides by column chromatography on Florisil (Mulhern et al., 1971), silica gel (Holden & Marsden 1969; Armour & Burke, 1970; Collins et al., 1972) or on charcoal (Berg et al., 1972; Jensen & Sundström, 1974). Several laboratories have reported difficulties in repeating results obtained by other investigators; the ease of separation appears to depend upon the characteristics of the absorbent, of the eluting solvent, and of the sample extract, though there appears to be no difficulty in separating all interfering substances except DDE, a metabolite of DDT. Thin-layer chromatography has been used for separation by Norén & Westöö (1968), Bagley et al. (1970), and Reinke et al. (1973).

In many environmental samples, DDE is present in large excess over the PCBs, and must be removed before the quantitative determination of PCBs. Oxidation procedures have been used to convert DDE to dichlorobenzophenone; recommended oxidants are potassium dichromate and sulfuric acid (Westöö & Norén, 1970b) and chromium (II) oxide and acetic acid (Mulhern et al., 1971). Jensen & Sundström (1974), who were interested in determining DDT/PCB ratios in environmental samples, preferred sodium dichromate in acetic acid with a trace of sulfuric acid. They claim that this does not destroy DDT and its metabolite DDD, which may be present in extracts after clean-up with strong sulfuric acid, and that using this mixture makes possible the quantitative determination of the dichlorobenzophenone from the oxidation of DDE.

Conversion of DDT to DDE may be achieved by treatment with ethanolic potassium hydroxide, which also removes interference from elemental sulfur (Ahling & Jensen, 1970). Sulfur may also be removed by activated Raney nickel (Ahnoff & Josefsson, 1975) or by metallic mercury.

Södergren (1973b) has scaled down the clean-up procedure for small samples, using microlitre volumes.

2.3.3 Chromatographic separation of PCBs

Gas–liquid chromatography

Most analysts use gas–liquid chromatography with an electron-capture detector for the separation of PCBs from the extract after clean-up. Stationary phases commonly used are silicones or their derivatives, for example, DC 200, SF 96, OV 1, and QF 1, or Apiezon L. Jensen & Sundström (1974) state that with a mixture of SF 96 and QF 1, 14 peaks can be obtained from Clophen A50, but that Apiezon L gives much better resolution. They obtained better peak separation by prior fractionation on a charcoal column, which separated the PCBs according to the number of *o*-chlorine substituents; they regard such refinements as unnecessary in PCB residue analysis, although they may be of value in the study of the selective, environmental degradation of PCBs. Column temperatures used ranged between 170°C and 230°C. Glass capillary columns gave good separation of PCBs from DDT and its metabolites (Schulte & Acker, 1974).

Thin-layer chromatography

This has been used in the clean-up stage, but it may also provide semi-quantitative results by visualization of the spots followed by densitometry, or by comparison with spots produced by known amounts of PCBs. Mulhern et al. (1971) separated PCBs on a plate coated with alumina containing silver nitrate, and the spots were developed by exposure to ultraviolet light; the detection limit was in the region of 1 μg. Collins et al. (1972) devised a similar method in which the PCBs remained together in a single spot, and they claimed a limit of detection of about 50 ng. Reversed-phase chromatography on plates coated with kieselguhr treated with liquid paraffin has been used to separate Phenochlor DP6 into several spots with a detection limit of a few micrograms (de Vos & Peet, 1971).

2.3.4 Quantification of PCB content

The response of the electron capture detector is not equal for all PCB components, being much affected by the degree of chlorination (Zitko et al., 1971). This does not lead to difficulties when the sample under investigation has been directly contaminated by a commercial PCB mixture, as that mixture can be used as a standard. Difficulties are encountered when the PCBs in the sample have undergone selective environmental degradation (see sections 3 and 5). Several investigators have noted that the pattern of peaks from such samples resembles fairly closely that of one or other of the higher chlorinated PCB mixtures such as Aroclor 1254, and they have compared the total area of the peaks with that of the nearest commercial product in order to determine the amount of PCBs in the sample (Armour & Burke, 1970). Collins et al. (1972) observed that, under their conditions, the area of peaks usually encountered in extracts of tissue samples was closely similar to that of an equivalent amount of DDE, thus DDE could be used for calibration. In order to overcome the uncertainties of these procedures, Rote & Murphy (1971) divided the peaks into groups according to the number of chlorine atoms in the molecule, as determined from mass spectrographic data, and calculated the PCB content of each group from the theoretical response of the detector to chlorine content. Jensen et al. (1973) selected a commercial PCB that included all the peaks from the extract; they determined the PCB content of each peak by combined mass spectrometry and coulometry, and determined the total PCBs in the sample by comparing the height of each peak obtained with the extract with those obtained with the reference sample. Simpler methods have been used by Koeman et al. (1969), who compared the height of a single peak obtained with the extract with that of a peak with the same retention time obtained with a commercial PCB mixture; others have averaged out more than one peak for this calculation (Reynolds, 1971; Reinke et al., 1973). Rote & Murphy (1971) have calculated that such procedures may more than double the values obtained by a more accurate method.

A different technique has been recommended by Berg et al. (1972); the PGBs are chlorinated with antimony pentachloride to decachlorobiphenyl, which can then be measured as a single peak.

2.3.5 Accuracy of PCB determinations

A group of eight analysts engaged in an investigation of pollution in the North Sea undertook a collaborative study to determine the PCB content of a sample of fish oil, using the methods currently employed in their laboratories (International Council for the Exploration of the Sea, 1974). The PCB values obtained ranged from 1.0 to 3.9 mg/kg with a mean of 1.97 mg/kg and a standard deviation of 0.93 mg/kg. Better agreement was obtained with the same fish oil fortified with PCBs at a concentration of 10 mg/kg; the mean of the results for the fortified sample was 10.0 mg/kg with a standard deviation of 1.1 mg/kg.

A probable source of error is incomplete initial extraction of PCBs from the sample (Holden & Marsden, 1969). Another source of variation between laboratories lies in the method used to quantify gas–liquid chromatographic peaks (section 2.3.4); van Hove Holdrinet (1975) considered this to be the major source of error.

It is evident that caution should be exercised in accepting the analytical results from a laboratory, particularly for samples with a low PCB content, until the competence of that laboratory has been established by an inter-laboratory collaborative study.

2.3.6   Confirmation of identity

Since Jensen first identified as PCBs those hitherto unknown substances that interfered in the gas–liquid chromatographic determination of organochlorine pesticides using mass spectrographic data, other investigators have confirmed the presence of PCBs in environmental samples by combining gas–liquid chromatography with mass spectrometry (Bagley et al., 1970) and with coulometry to measure the chlorine content. The conversion of PCBs to bicyclohexyl and decachlorobiphenyl is further confirmation (Berg et al., 1972). The widespread distribution of PCBs is now well established, and, as adequate methods are available to remove interference from organochlorine pesticides, there is no evidence of the presence of other interfering substances in the types of sample that have so far been analysed, down to a limit of detection of around 0.01 mg/kg. This does not necessarily apply to other types of sample, particularly when very low levels are being sought; Ahnoff & Josefsson (1973, 1975) reported a number of unknown interfering substances, when measuring PCBs in water at levels below 1 ng/litre, one of which was subsequently identified as elemental sulfur. They recommend confirmation by mass fragmentography for such samples.

2.4   Determination of PCTs

A few methods have been published for the determination of PCTs; extraction and clean-up procedures are similar to those used for PCBs, but the gas–liquid chromatographic details are different because of the lower volatility of the PCTs. Zitko et al. (1972b) used 3% OV 210 as the stationary phase with a column temperature of 200°C. Thomas & Reynolds (1973) also used OV 210 with a column temperature of 250°C and another system with 3% Dexsil as stationary phase at 300°C with a ^{63}Ni electron capture detector; this was also used by Addison et al. (1972). Sosa-Lucero et al. (1973) used OV 210 and SE 30 at 255°C and Freudental & Greve (1973) used OV 17 with a temperature programmed from 200°C to 285°C. Thomas & Reynolds (1973) confirmed the identity by chlorination to tetradecachloroterphenyl with antimony pentachloride.

A thin-layer chromatographic technique has also been described with a limit of detection of about 1 µg (Addison et al., 1972).

3. SOURCES OF ENVIRONMENTAL POLLUTION

3.1 Production and Uses of PCBs

Details of the production and uses of PCBs in the USA have been released, and have been summarized by Nisbet & Sarofim (1972). Annual production has increased steadily since 1930 and reached a maximum in 1970 of 33 000 tonnes. During this peak year, 65% of the production was of the 42% chlorinated type, 25% was less chlorinated, and the remainder more chlorinated. After 1970, production sharply decreased owing to voluntary limitation of sales by the Monsanto Company, the sole manufacturer in the USA. According to information collected by the Organization for Economic Co-operation and Development (OECD), the 1971 production in the USA was 18 000 tonnes and the total in OECD countries in that year was 48 000 tonnes. It has been estimated that the cumulative total production of PCBs in North America up to 1971 was 0.5 million tonnes, and in the whole world probably double this figure.

The commercial applications of PCBs have been reviewed in an OECD report (Organization for Economic Co-operation and Development, 1973). From an environmental viewpoint these can be divided into three categories:

Controllable closed systems. PCBs used as dielectrics in transformers and large capacitors have a life equal to that of the equipment, and with proper design leakage does not occur. When the equipment is scrapped the quantity of dielectric is sufficiently large to justify regeneration.

Uncontrollable closed systems. PCBs are used in heat transfer and hydraulic systems which, although technically closed, permit leakage. The need for frequent replacement of small quantities makes recovery impracticable. PCBs are very widely dispersed in small capacitors, and there are great difficulties in collecting these items for disposal.

Dissipative uses. PCBs have been used in the formulation of lubricating and cutting oils, in pesticides, and as plasticizers in paints, copying paper, adhesives, sealants, and plastics. In these applications, the PCBs are in direct contact with the environment, and there is no way of recovering them when the product is scrapped.

The uses of PCBs in the USA in 1970 have been analysed by Nisbet & Sarofim (1972). Of the total 33 000 tonnes, 56% was used as a dielectric, with 36% in capacitors and 20% in transformers. Various plasticizer outlets accounted for 30%, hydraulic fluids and lubricants 12%, and heat transfer liquids 1.5%. Following the restriction of sales for non-dissipative uses, the percentage of PCBs sold as dielectrics rose to 77% in 1971 and the proportion of highly chlorinated products was considerably reduced, Aroclor 1016 replacing Aroclor 1242. In Japan, 44 800 tonnes of PCBs were used from 1962 to 1971, and of this 65.4% was used in the electrical industry, 11.3% in heat exchangers, 17.9% in pressure-sensitive duplicating paper, and 5.4% for other dissipative uses (Ishi, 1972). In Sweden, most of the 600 tonnes imported in 1969 was used in the electrical industry and a large part of the remainder in paints (Jensen, unpublished report 1972).

According to the OECD report, transformers and capacitors provided the major outlets for PCBs in most OECD countries in 1971. In 1972, several countries restricted sales; in Sweden the importation and use of PCBs were restricted by law; in the United Kingdom, as in the USA, sales were voluntarily restricted to the lower chlorinated PCBs for use as dielectrics in enclosed systems; in the Federal Republic of Germany, use in hydraulic and heat transfer fluids was also permitted. In Japan the production and use of PCBs were banned in 1972. Limitations on sales were subsequently introduced in other countries.

No information is available on the scale of production and the uses of PCTs.

3.2 Entry of PCBs into the Environment

Surveys of the sources of environmental pollution with PCBs were made before production and use were limited, and the information available may not now apply in North America and elsewhere. Table 4 gives an estimate of the fate of the PCBs produced in 1970 in the USA (Nisbet & Sarofim, 1972). Only 20% of the annual production can be regarded as a net increase in current usage, and the remainder is balanced by a loss to the environment. More than one-half of this entered dumps and landfills and it has been calculated that 0.3 million tonnes of PCBs have accumulated in such locations in North America since 1930. Much of this was originally enclosed in containers such as capacitors or was in plasticized resins and will not be released until the containing medium decays. The diffusion of PCBs from landfills is likely to be slow on account of their low volatility and low water solubility; Carnes et al. (1973) found little leaching from one site they tested.

Table 4. Entry of PCBs into the environment[a]

Route	Percentage of annual production	PCB type (% chlorination)
Vaporization from plasticizers	4.5	48–60
Vaporization during incineration	1	42
Leaks and disposal of industrial fluids	13	42–60
Destruction by incineration	9	mainly 42
Disposal in dumps and landfills	52.5	42–60
Net increase in current usage	20	42–54

[a] From Nisbet & Sarofim, 1972.

Pollution of the environment has occurred mainly from the first three routes mentioned in Table 4. In addition, there are other routes, which although involving relatively small amounts, nevertheless have an influence on the entry of PCBs into food chains. PCBs have been used in the USA in amounts of about 10 tonnes/year in pesticide formulations (Panel on Hazardous Trace Substances, 1972), and the unauthorized use of scrap transformer fluid for this purpose has led to local contamination of milk supplies.

Pressure sensitive duplicating paper containing PCBs has found its way into waste paper supplies and has been recycled into paper and board used as food packaging materials; paints for coating the bottom of ships contained 3–5% of PCBs—about 3% of the annual quantity imported into Sweden has been used for this purpose—and this has been a source of plankton contamination (Jensen et al., 1972a).

3.2.1 Release of PCBs into the atmosphere

There appears to be little widespread atmospheric contamination during the manufacture and processing of PCBs, but this can occur during their subsequent use and disposal. Although PCBs have a low volatility, there may be an appreciable loss to the atmosphere during the lifetime of a PCB-plasticized resin, particularly of the lower chlorinated products. Further pollution may occur during the incineration of industrial and municipal waste. Most municipal incinerators are not very effective in destroying PCBs; efficient incinerators can be designed for this purpose (Jensen & Wickberg, unpublished report 1971; Jensen, unpublished report 1972), although the higher chlorinated PCBs are more resistant to pyrolysis. Secondary sources of atmospheric pollution are volatilization from soil, and from the drying of sewage sludge. Laveskog (1973) found that the PCB emissions from municipal incineration and from the drying of sewage sludge each amounted to about 1 kg/year per million inhabitants, a small amount compared with the 2 tonnes deposited yearly from aerial fallout in the south of Sweden.

3.2.2 Leakage and disposal of PCBs in industry

The major source of environmental pollution with PCBs, which eventually affects food chains, is the leakage and the disposal of industrial fluids. There have been serious cases of poisoning in man (Kuratsune et al., 1972) and in animals (Panel on Hazardous Trace Substances, 1972) due to leakage from a heat exchanger. Leakages, or the unintentional or deliberate discharge of waste, have contaminated seas, lakes, waterways, and sewers (Duke et al., 1970; Schmidt et al., 1971; Veith, 1972).

Analysis of solids from factory wastes in Japan have revealed a wide variation in PCB content. In most, less than 1 mg/kg was detected, but in some the contamination was very heavy, the highest level recorded being 8.26% from a factory manufacturing electrical equipment (Japanese Environment & Safety Bureau, unpublished report 1972).

4. ENVIRONMENTAL TRANSPORT AND TRANSFORMATION

4.1 Environmental Transport

Nisbet & Sarofim (1972) emphasize that the available data are insufficient to determine anything but a very crude model of the transfer of PCBs into the environment. Guesses can be made by referring to the distribution of DDT, which resembles the PCBs to some extent in its physical and chemical properties and about which more is known. Much of the following discussion arises from their analysis of the situation in the North American continent.

4.1.1 Air transport

By analogy with DDT, it might be expected that PCBs entering the atmosphere in the vapour phase would be adsorbed rapidly on to particles, which would be deposited or washed out in rain at a rate depending on their particle size, the average residence time in the atmosphere being 2–3 days. This has been confirmed by Södergren (1972a), who measured the deposition in southern Sweden of PCBs that had originated from municipal incinerators or had been carried over from Denmark by the prevailing winds, and showed that the amount deposited in central Sweden was much less. Carnes (1973) and Laveskog, (unpublished report 1973) found mainly particulate PCBs in the emission from incinerators. Harvey & Steinhauer (1974), however, considered that the results of their analyses of air in north Atlantic regions indicated that most of the PCBs carried in the air were in the vapour phase.

4.1.2 Transport in soil

The PCBs in soil are derived mainly from particulate deposition, estimated at 1000–2000 tonnes annually in North America, most of which is in urban areas. Small amounts have originated from the use of sewage sludge as a fertilizer, from the leaching of landfills, and from the use of PCBs in pesticide formulations. Tucker et al. (1975) found that under experimental conditions, the higher chlorinated PCBs were not leached from soils by percolating water, and those with a lower level of chlorination were removed only slowly, particularly from soils of high clay content. Losses do occur by volatilization and by biotransformation; by analogy with DDT and its metabolites the half-time in soil has been estimated at 5 years. Haque et al. (1974) showed that the rate of evaporation decreased with the clay content of the soil and the degree of chlorination of the biphenyl, and increased with temperature. Biotransformation has also been shown to play a part in the disappearance of the lower chlorinated compounds from soil (Iwata et al., 1973).

The total amount of PCBs distributed over North America, apart from that in dumps and landfills, has been estimated at 20 000 tonnes, of which one quarter has subsequently been transported via the air to the seas. (Nisbet & Sarofim, 1972).

4.1.3 Transport in water

The entry of PCBs into water occurs mainly at the points of discharge of industrial and urban wastes into rivers, lakes, and coastal waters. Sewage treatment appears to remove particulate PCBs from water, but not PCBs in solution; these are concentrated in the sludge (Ahling & Jensen, 1970), which may be dumped into rivers and coastal waters. Holden (1970b) found a mean PCB content of 3 mg/kg in liquid sludges from Glasgow, and calculated that PCBs at the rate of 1 tonne/year were released into the Clyde and Thames estuaries; a similar output was calculated from water treatment plants off the California coast (Schmidt et al., 1971). Other localized sources of pollution are leakages or waste disposal from ships. PCBs in water are attached mainly to particulate matter (Södergren, 1973a) and eventually fall to the bottom sediment at a rate that depends on the particle size. PCBs may be leached from the sediment and may reach coastal waters, but Nimmo et al. (1971) noted little change in the PCB content of a sediment at a point downstream from a source of contamination over a period of 9 months. The process may be accelerated by the dumping of dredging spoil.

4.1.4 Transport through biota

According to the approximate calculations of Nisbet & Sarofim (1972), less than 1000 tonnes of PCBs are located in living organisms throughout the world, so that biological transport and degradation play little part in the fate of PCBs in the environment, though these factors have great ecotoxicological significance.

4.2 Transformation in the Environment

4.2.1 Abiotic transformation

The fate of the various PCBs in commercial mixtures depends on their physical and chemical properties. Some fractionation occurs during the volatilization of PCBs, because of a decrease in vapour pressure with increasing chlorination. The PCBs are chemically very stable, and are not likely to be degraded at a significant rate by hydrolytic or similar reactions under environmental conditions. They are, however, fairly easily degraded by photolysis under laboratory conditions; Safe & Hutzinger (1971), and Hutzinger et al. (1972b) have shown that PCBs are dechlorinated in hexane solution at a rate that increases with increasing chlorination. PCBs in aqueous-dioxane suspensions and in thin films give hydroxy and carboxylic acid derivatives on irradiation. The lower chlorinated biphenyls, at a vapour concentration in air of 1.5 mg/m^3 are readily destroyed by photolysis under laboratory conditions. There is no direct evidence of the extent of PCB breakdown in the atmosphere under environmental conditions, and nothing is known of the persistence and toxicity of any transformation products.

4.2.2 Biotransformation

The biotransformation of PCBs is discussed in section 6.6. Owing to the small proportion of the total environmental PCBs contained in living matter, biotransformation does not significantly influence the overall

31

environmental concentrations of PCBs, though it has a marked influence on PCBs passing through food chains.

4.2.3 Metabolism in limited ecosystems

The presence of PCBs in sewage sludge suggests that they are not all readily transformed by microorganisms. Choi et al. (1974) found no evidence of biotransformation of Aroclor 1254 added to water entering an aerated biological water treatment system, although much of it was removed with the sludge; there appeared to be no interference by the PCBs in the performance of the system. Vodden (1973) quotes investigations showing that PCBs with four or fewer chlorine atoms are readily broken down by microorganisms, but that this can be inhibited by the presence of higher chlorinated PCBs. Mono- and dichlorobiphenyl can be transformed by *Achromobacter* isolated from sewage effluent (Ahmed & Focht, 1973), and a culture of lake bacteria can degrade some of the lower chlorinated components of Aroclor 1242 to chlorine-free derivatives (Kaiser & Wong, 1974).

Södergren (1972b) investigated the transport of Clophen A50 added to a model aquatic ecosystem; this was rapidly taken up by an alga (*Chlorella*) and no change was observed in the proportion of the component PCBs in the first consumer fish; however, there was a relative loss of the lower chlorinated PCBs in the perch, the second consumer. No progressive loss of the lower chlorinated PCBs was observed in sediment, plankton, invertebrates, and fish inhabiting a Swedish lake (Södergren, 1973a). Evidence on the metabolism of PCBs by fish is conflicting, but it seems probable that most fish, particularly those in the lower trophic stages of food chains, cannot readily degrade the low chlorinated PCBs.

4.3 Biological Accumulation

Although PCB concentrations in living organisms clearly indicate a progressive accumulation in food chains, the factors discussed in the previous sections make it impossible to give any reliable figure for bioaccumulation at each trophic stage. There is also doubt about which tissue level should be used in the calculation, that of the whole body, the fat, or the liver.

There is good evidence that all aquatic organisms studied in aquaria can absorb PCBs directly from water. The accumulation varies with the duration of exposure and the concentration in the ambient water. A diatom exposed to Aroclor 1242 showed an accumulation factor of 1100

(Keil et al., 1971); with Aroclor 1254 the following values have been obtained: pink shrimp, 6600; blue crab, 4600; oyster, 8100; pinfish, 980 (Duke et al., 1970); spot, 37 000 (Hansen et al., 1971); bluegills, up to 71 400 (Stalling & Mayer, 1972). The accumulation factor in scud exposed to Aroclor 1254 reached a maximum of 24 000 within 4 days and thereafter remained fairly constant (Sanders & Chandler, 1972). Similar results were obtained with other invertebrates, although with crayfish the uptake was slower and the accumulation was still increasing after 21 days. However, it is probable that most of the PCBs entering aquatic systems are retained by particulate matter, and the above accumulation factors are not necessarily applicable to natural ecosystems. Nimmo et al. (1971) demonstrated that the fiddler crab could ingest PCB contained in the bottom sediment. When exposed to Aroclor 1254 in water, ciliated protozoa, stated to be the major benthic input to aquatic food chains, had an accumulation factor of 60 (Cooley et al., 1972).

5. ENVIRONMENTAL LEVELS AND EXPOSURES

5.1 Air

Mean concentrations in air, in several locations in Sweden, ranged from the detection limit of 0.8 ng/m^3–3.9 ng/m^3. The highest figure recorded was 12.5 ng/m^3 (Ekstedt & Odén, 1974). In the USA, PCB concentrations in air ranged from 5 ng/m^3 near the north-east coast to 0.05 ng/m^3 at a distance of 2000 m out over the Atlantic Ocean (Harvey & Steinhauer, 1974). Results from the United States Environmental Protection Agency indicate a range between 1 and 50 ng/m^3 (Panel on Hazardous Trace Substances, 1972), and similar results have been reported from Japan (Tatsukawa & Watanabe, 1972).

5.2 Soil and Sediments

In Sweden, PCBs have been found in natural soil at a concentration of 15 µg/kg by Odén & Berggren (1973). The same authors also found 0.006–1.4 mg/kg in sediments from areas in the Baltic Sea with different degrees of pollution. Nimmo et al. (1971) found PCB levels of 1.4–61 mg/kg in sediment from an estuary at a point near the site of an accidental release of PCBs from a factory, and levels of 0.6 mg/kg at a point 16 km downstream. Soil samples from the bank 6.5 km downstream from the source contained 1.4–1.7 mg/kg. Less than 1 mg/kg has been found in Japanese agricultural soil, but as much as 510 mg/kg in soil near a factory making electrical components (Fukada, et al., 1973).

5.3 Water

In heavily contaminated waters, PCB concentrations may be several times greater than their solubility, owing to adsorption on suspended particles (Duke et al., 1970). Water in a Swedish river contained 0.5 ng/litre as it entered a water treatment plant, and 0.33 ng/litre in the tap water produced (Ahling & Jensen, 1970). Values of 0.1–0.3 ng/litre have been measured in other Swedish rivers (Ahnoff & Josefsson, 1974). Södergren (1973a) found a seasonal variation in the PCB level in a Swedish lake, with a maximum of 2 ng/litre, the pollution being attributed to aerial fallout. Concentrations of 10–100 ng/litre have been measured in tap water at Kyoto in Japan (Panel on Hazardous Trace Substances, 1972). In a polluted coastal area of Lake Michigan in 1970, PCB concentrations of from 450 to less than 100 ng/litre were measured in 1970, but there was a marked decrease in 1971, possibly due to the limitation on sales of PCBs (Panel on Hazardous Trace Substances, 1972). From the scanty information on PCBs, reinforced by analogy with the more extensive information on DDT, it has been estimated that nonpolluted fresh waters should contain not more than 0.5 ng/litre up to 5 ng/litre for the Great Lakes of North America, 50 ng/litre for moderately polluted rivers and estuaries, and 500 ng/litre for highly polluted rivers.

5.4 Living Organisms

There is now considerable information from Canada, Japan, Sweden, the United Kingdom, and the USA, on the accumulation of PCB's in biological material. Analytical measurements on different organisms, and on the same organism from different localities, vary widely and it is necessary to consider the factors that lead to this variation. Differences in analytical techniques may contribute to this (see section 2.3.5) but important influences are exerted by the extent of local pollution, the amount of fat in the organism studied, and its trophic stage in food chains.

5.4.1 The influence of local pollution

Most of the fish eaten by man is taken from waters with relatively little pollution. In a collaborative study by seven national laboratories

(International Council for the Exploration of the Sea, 1974), the PCB content of muscle tissue of fish taken from the North Sea was measured. A mean of 0.01 mg/kg was found in cod, herring contained up to 0.48 mg/kg with most samples in the range of 0.1–0.2 mg/kg, and plaice contained 0.1 mg/kg or less. Similar values were reported by Zitko (1971) for fish taken from the North Atlantic.

There are many examples of different PCB levels in similar species collected from areas of high and low pollution. Jensen, et al. (1972b) found five times as much PCBs in herrings caught in waters off industrialized areas near Stockholm, as in herrings from the cleaner waters of the west coast of Sweden. Similarly, levels in plankton harvested along the Swedish archipelago at various distances from Stockholm fell progressively, away from the more polluted areas (Jensen, et al., 1972c); the concentration in pike fell to one-half (Olsson & Jensen, 1974). Koeman et al., (1972b) found PCB levels of up to 88 mg/kg in the blubber of toothed whales caught in the North Sea, but none was detectable in similar species from New Zealand or Surinam. Holden (1973b) found high PCB concentrations in the blubber of seals in polluted coastal areas of the United Kingdom (up to 235 mg/kg), and much lower levels in unpolluted areas (down to 2 mg/kg).

Risebrough & de Lappe (1972) studied the PCB content of extractable lipids from brown pelican eggs collected from areas throughout North and South America, and showed that the content varied from 4 mg/kg up to 266 mg/kg in highly industrialized regions. They also reported levels greater than 3 mg/kg in fish from New York Sound and Tokyo Bay, both very polluted areas. Even higher levels of PCBs have been found in fish from polluted lakes and inland waterways, a level of 20 mg/kg being found in fish from Lake Ontario, and over 200 mg/kg in fish from the Hudson River (Stalling & Mayer, 1972). Similar correlations between pollution and PCB levels have been reported from the United Kingdom in fish (Portmann, 1970), and in mussels (Holdgate, 1971).

The association between high PCB levels and local pollution may be disturbed by the migratory habits of certain species, particularly in birds that may be exposed to PCBs in their wintering areas or on the migration routes. As much as 400 mg/kg has been measured in the fat of a robin entering Sweden, although the normal value is about 16 mg/kg. Many migratory birds start egg-laying on arrival at their summer quarters, so the PCB content of eggs may reflect the bird's previous exposure rather than the local pollution (Odsjö, 1973). A special case concerning the effect of pollution is seen in the use of fish-feed in poultry and fish farming. Kolbye (1972) stated that this may contain PCB levels of 0.6–4.5 mg/kg.

5.4.2　The influence of the fat content of tissues

PCBs are mainly stored in body fat (see section 5.5.5.1), and the total PCB content of the body tissues is much influenced by their fat content (Portmann, 1970; Westöö & Norén, 1970a). Jensen, et al. (1969) found PCB levels of 0.27 mg/kg and 0.33 mg/kg respectively, in the muscle tissue of herring and cod from the same area of the Baltic, although the cod is at a higher trophic stage (see section 5.4.3). These two species have 4.4 and 0.32% of extractable fat respectively, and when the PCB level is calculated on the fat content, values of 6.8 mg/kg for the herring and 11 mg/kg for the cod are obtained. Cod liver has a much higher fat content than cod muscle and Jensen (1973) has reported the ratio of PCB concentrations in cod liver and muscle to be over 100, the maximum in liver being 59 mg/kg. Jensen et al. (1969) have remarked that the considerable seasonal variation in the fat content of the herring, rising from 1% in spring to 10% in autumn, influences the tissue level of PCBs. Peakall et al. (1972) noticed a marked rise in tissue levels in starved birds owing to the mobilization of fat, and it is possible that the high levels of PCBs in the livers of birds dying during the "seabird wreck" in the Irish Sea were secondary to emaciation (Holdgate, 1971). De Freitas & Norstrom (1974) showed that, in pigeons, pure PCBs left fatty tissues and accumulated mainly in muscle during the mobilization of fat associated with starvation.

5.4.3　The influence of the trophic stage in food

Swedish work on the distribution of PCBs in aquatic ecosystems has been summarized by Jensen et al. (1972b), and Olsson et al. (1973), and it has been largely confirmed by work in other areas (Risebrough et al., 1968; Risebrough & de Lappe, 1972: Holdgate, 1971). Zoo- and phyto-plankton readily absorb or adsorb PCBs from their environment; Söder-gren (1972) has demonstrated the rapid uptake of Clophen A50 by the unicellular alga *Chlorella*. Marine zooplankton may contain PCB levels of 5 mg/kg in extractable lipids in areas of moderate pollution (Jensen et al., 1972c; Williams & Holden, 1973), with somewhat lower values in rela-tively unpolluted areas. However, results with plankton, particularly where high levels are found, must be regarded with caution as the sample could be contaminated with PCB-rich oil or tar particles. Herring feeding on plankton in areas of moderate pollution contain PCB levels of about 0.5 mg/kg in muscle tissue (10 mg/kg in extractable fat); plaice and flounder, both bottom-feeding fish contain about one-third of this, presumably because the PCB content of benthic organisms is lower. In predatory fish such as the cod and pike, the PCB level in extractable fat is about 10 mg/kg and a mean of 10 mg/kg has been measured in the blubber of seals.

Much higher PCB values have been obtained in fish-eating birds; levels of 18 mg/kg (650 mg/kg in extractable fat), and 17 mg/kg (420 mg/kg in extractable fat) were found in the herring gull and comorant respectively. Lower values were found in birds feeding on invertebrates, such as the long-tailed duck which contained 14 mg/kg in fat; marine invertebrates contain PCB levels in the region of 0.1–0.2 mg/kg. At the top trophic level, 96 mg/kg (9.7 g/kg in extractable fat) has been measured in the eagle owl; the highest recorded PCB values were from eagle owls found dead in the south-east coastal region of Sweden, 260 mg/kg in the brain (3.4 g/kg in extractable fat) and 110 mg/kg in muscle (12 g/kg in extractable fat). (Odsjö, 1973).

Less information is available on terrestrial ecosystems. PCB concentrations in the region of 0.01 mg/kg have been found in fresh tissue in slugs, snakes, and ants, and slightly higher concentrations in earthworms. Tissue levels were generally at the limit of detection (0.01 mg/kg) in herbivorous mammals (Odsjö, 1973). Brüggemann et al. (1974) reported a mean PCB concentration of 0.22 mg/kg in 20 out of 72 measurements in the adipose tissues of the hare and a higher value (2.5 mg/kg) in 1 out of 5 tests on the adipose tissues of the fox. Higher values have been found in the American mink in Sweden with 0.58 mg/kg in muscle (45 mg/kg in fat) presumably because of a fish diet (Odsjö, 1973). Tissue levels in wild birds on a mixed diet are variable and rather low, but those in predatory birds are higher. Prestt et al. (1970) related the PCB concentration in the liver of wild birds to their diet; less than 1 mg/kg was found in insectivorous birds and more than 70 mg/kg in the sparrow hawk. A level of 0.5 mg/kg has been found in the muscle of the eagle owl in central Sweden, but this is much less than the tissue concentrations encountered in this bird in coastal areas (Odsjö, 1973). High tissue concentrations in predatory and marine birds have also been reported from Canada (Gilbertson & Reynolds, 1974), the Netherlands (Koeman et al., 1972a), and from the United Kingdom (Bourne & Bogan, 1972).

5.4.4 Indicator organisms

Several of the organisms, that have been shown to accumulate PCBs from the environment, have been suggested as indicators of the extent of local pollution with PCBs. In aquatic systems, the use of plankton as an indicator has the advantage that it is at the lowest trophic stage of food chains but errors may occur in the determination because of the inclusion in the sample of nonplanktonic particles with a high PCB content (Jensen et al., 1972a). The herring, which feeds on plankton, has been suggested as an indicator (Jensen et al., 1972b) and, at higher trophic stages, the pike, which is a stationary fish (Olsson & Jensen, unpublished report, 1974), and seabirds (Jensen et al., 1972c). In fresh waters, the amphipod *Gammarus pulex* has been used as an indicator organism for chlorinated hydrocarbons (Södergren et al., 1972). However, Zitko et al. (1974) claimed that the variation between individual fish was so high that Atlantic herring and yellow perch could be used to detect trends in pollution only if large numbers were taken for analysis, with an interval between measurements of at least 4 years.

A series of monitoring studies has been made by OECD, the species selected covering terrestial, fresh water, and marine environments. The analytical results, and the general problems of selecting species for monitoring, have been discussed by Holden. (1970a, 1973a, 1973b).

5.5   The Extent of Human Exposure to PCBs and PCTs

5.5.1   Air and water

The maximum concentration of PCBs in air is not likely to exceed 50 ng/m^3 (section 5.1). The highest concentration of PCBs reported in domestic tap water is 100 ng/litre in the Kyoto area of Japan (Panel on Hazardous Trace Substances, 1972), but levels more likely to be encountered should not exceed 1 ng/litre (section 5.3).

5.5.2   Food

The PCB content of a variety of foods on the Swedish market has been measured by Westöö & Norén (1970a) and Westöö et al. (1971). Less than 0.1 mg/kg was found in samples of butter, margarine, vegetable oils, eggs, beef, lamb, chicken, bread, biscuits, and baby food; one sample of pork out of more than 100 had a PCB content in the range of 0.2–0.5 mg/kg. As might be expected from the discussion in section 5.4, higher values were found in fish depending on the fat content and the pollution of the fishing area (Westöö & Norén, 1970a; Berglund, 1972). The PCB levels obtained in an extensive study by the US Food and Drug Administration are shown in Table 5.

These values are considerably higher than those reported from Sweden but they are probably biased, as they include samples originating from areas previously suspected of having been subject to local pollution. In a

Canadian survey, PCB levels of less than 0.01 mg/kg were found in eggs (Mes et al., 1974) and a mean of 0.042 mg/kg was found in domestic and imported cheese with a maximum of 0.27 mg/kg (Villeneuve et al., 1973b). No traces of PCTs were found.

In Japan, a similar range of PCB contents for most foods has been reported; however, some high levels have been reported for rice and vegetables harvested in fields polluted with PCBs (Environmental Sanitation Bureau, 1973). The PCB content of most fish on the market was less than 3 mg/kg, although some contained more than this. The PCT content of fish was much lower (Fukano et al., 1974). In the Netherlands, eel has been reported to contain PCT levels of 0.2–0.5 mg/kg and PCB levels of 4.7 mg/kg (Freudenthal & Greve, 1973).

Table 5. PCB levels in food in the USA[a]

Food	% positive (0.1 mg/kg)	Level in positive samples (mg/kg) Mean	Maximum
Cheese	6	0.25	1.0
Milk	7	2.3	27.8
Eggs	29	0.55	3.7
Fish	54	1.87	35.3

[a] From Kolbye (1972).

Samples of butter from the Westphalian area of the Federal Republic of Germany, obtained in the period 1972–74, contained PCB levels of 0.38 mg/kg (range 0.25–0.54 mg/kg) (Claus & Acker, 1975).

Relatively high PCB levels in some packaged foods in Sweden, mainly of imported origin, could be attributed to migration from the packaging material (Westöö et al., 1971). The highest level encountered was 11 mg/kg in a children's breakfast cereal; PCB levels of 70 mg/kg and 700 mg/kg were found in the material of the inner bag containing this product and in the outer cardboard container respectively. Up to 2000 mg/kg was found in cartons of other samples. Villeneuve et al. (1973a) have analysed packaged food in Canada; they found that 66.7% of the samples contained PCB levels of less than 0.01 mg/kg, 30.7% contained between 0.01 and 1 mg/kg, and 2.6% contained more than 1 mg/kg. PCT determinations were also made on these samples; 94.5% of the samples contained less than 0.01 mg/kg and 5.5% contained 0.01–0.05 mg/kg. The highest PCB levels were encountered in a rice sample with 2.1 mg/kg where the packaging material contained 31 mg/kg, and in a dried fruit sample with 4.5 mg/kg in a container containing 76 mg/kg. In a survey of packaging containers, approximately 80% were found to contain PCB and PCT levels of less than 1 mg/kg, while about 4% contained levels higher than 10 mg/kg. The most likely source of PCBs in packaging materials is the recycling of paper waste containing pressure-sensitive duplicating paper (Masuda et al., 1972).

5.5.3 Occupational exposure

Occupational exposure does not only occur during the manufacture of PCBs and with their use in the electrical industry. It may also be wide-spread among mechanics in contact with lubricating oils and hydraulic fluids, among workers exposed to varnishes and paints, and among office workers from contact with pressure-sensitive duplicating paper, some brands of which readily transfer PCBs to skin (Kuratsune & Masuda, 1972b). Studies in Finland showed that whole blood from persons with no special exposure to PCBs contained 0.3–1.2 μg/100 ml, while blood from persons handling PCBs in an analytical laboratory contained 3.6–6.3 μg/100 ml and blood from workers in a capacitor factory had PCB levels of 7.5–190 μg/100 ml in the blood and 30–700 mg/kg in fat. No signs of toxicity were evident in these workers (Karppanen & Kolho, 1973). Similar plasma values were found in workers from Japanese capacitor factories, but here skin lesions were noted (Hasegawa et al., 1972a). This same study reported that air levels of PCBs of 0.01–0.05 mg/m^3 were measured in a factory where KC-300 was used in the manufacture of electric condensers. PCB levels in serum in workers ranged from 10 to 65 μg/100 ml.[a] One month after the use of PCBs had been suspended, serum levels still ranged from 9 to 74 μg/100 ml. However, in another factory making electric condensers, serum levels decreased from an average of 80 μg/100 ml to 30 μg/100 ml within three months of the use of PCBs being suspended (Kitamura et al., 1973). According to Hara et al. (1974), the half-time of PCBs in the blood of workers engaged in the manufacture of electric condensers for less than 5 years was several months, while that of workers employed for more than 10 years was 2–3 years. Hammer et al. (1972) found a higher frequency of measurable plasma values in workers working with refuse burners than in a control group.

5.5.4 Other sources of exposure

Broadhurst (1972) has reviewed the many technical applications of PCBs that appear in the literature and in patent specifications, and which

---

[a] In this document, the concentrations of PCBs in blood and serum are expressed in μg/100 ml although in some original papers the values are given in μg/100 g. For practical purposes the differences, about 5% and 3% respectively, can be neglected.

indicate the possibility of a widespread nonoccupational low-level exposure to PCBs, other than that deriving from the diet. PCBs are used in the home in ballast capacitors for fluorescent lighting, and exposure deriving from pressure-sensitive copying paper has not been limited to office workers. The valuable properties of PCBs as plasticizers has led to their use in furnishings, interior decoration, and building construction; examples are surface treatment for textiles, adhesive for waterproof wall coatings, paints, and sealant putties. PCBs have been used as plasticizers for plastic materials and in the formulation of printing inks.

5.5.5 Biological indices of human exposure

The only surveys of value have been on body fat, blood, and milk.

5.5.5.1 *Body fat*

In a survey of 637 fat samples taken at autopsy or during surgery in the USA, 68.9% contained PCB levels of less than 1 mg/kg, 25.9% contained 1–2 mg/kg, and 5.2% contained more than 2 mg/kg (Yobs, 1972). A similar distribution was found in a smaller survey by Price & Welch (1972). In the Kochi area of Japan, a mean PCB level of 2.86 mg/kg was recorded with an upper limit of 7.5 mg/kg; about double these values were found in the Kyoto area (Nishimoto et al., 1972a, 1972b). Bjerk (1972) reported average PCB levels of 0.9 mg/kg (1.6 mg/kg on a lipid basis) in adipose tissue, taken at 40 autopsies in the Oslo area. Curley et al. (1973b) found PCB levels ranging from 0.30 to 1.48 mg/kg in a total of 241 human adipose samples in Japan. A mean value of 5.7 mg/kg has been reported for 20 samples from the Federal Republic of Germany (Acker & Schulte, 1970); in a more recent study, 282 adipose tissue samples from different areas were found to contain PCB levels of 8.3 mg/kg of adipose tissue on a lipid basis (Acker & Schulte, 1974). In Austria, a range of PCB levels of 0.3–7.3 mg/kg on a lipid weight basis was found in 32 residents in the Vienna metropolitan area; an increase of the PCB concentration with age was not observed (Pesendorfer et al., 1973). Detectable levels of PCBs were found in only a few of 201 human fat samples in the United Kingdom and in these, the level did not exceed 1 mg/kg (Abbott et al., 1972). A survey of 51 human fat samples in New Zealand showed that all samples contained PCB residues with an average of 0.82 mg/kg (Solly & Shanks, 1974).

Doguchi et al. (1974) found an average PCT level of 0.6 mg/kg in human fat with a range of 0.1–2.1 mg/kg. Takizawa & Minagawa (1974) also found PCT levels of 0.02 mg/kg in human liver ($n=6$), 0.01 mg/kg in the kidney ($n=2$), 0.02 mg/kg in the brain ($n=3$) and 0.04 mg/kg in the pancreas ($n = 1$). In the Netherlands, PCTs were found in human fat at levels of 0–1 mg/kg (Freudenthal & Greve, 1973).

5.5.5.2 *Blood*

43% of blood plasma samples from 723 volunteers in the USA showed the presence of PCBs; the mean value in these was about 0.5 μg/100 ml (Finklea et al., 1972). Studies in Finland on whole blood showed 0.31–1.2 μg/100 ml in persons with no special exposure to PCBs (Karppanen & Kolho, 1973). In Japan, an average PCB level of 0.32 μg/100 ml and a PCT level of 0.5 μg/100 ml have been recorded in the blood of non-occupationally exposed volunteers (Doguchi & Fukano, 1975). In patients with severe weight loss, high levels of PCBs in the blood (up to 10 μg/100 ml) were noted (Hesselberg & Scherr, 1974). This was attributed to the release of PCBs from the mobilization of fat.

5.5.5.3 *Human milk*

PCB concentrations measured in whole human milk in Sweden were 0.014 mg/litre in 1967 and 0.025 mg/litre in 1971–72 (Westöö & Norén, 1972), 0.03 mg/litre in Japan (Nishimoto et al., 1972a), 0.103 in the Federal Republic of Germany (Acker & Schulte, 1970) and 0.02 mg/litre in Canada (Musial et al., 1974). A survey in Colorado, USA, revealed 8 positive samples out of 39, within the range of 0.04–0.1 mg/kg (Savage et al., 1973).

5.5.6 Estimated daily intake

From the PCB levels encountered in air and drinking water (section 5.5.1), the daily intake from each of these sources is likely to be less than 1 μg.

It has been stated that the major part of the human dietary intake of PCBs is from fish (Berglund, 1972; Hammond, 1972). This may well be true in areas such as Japan or certain localities near the North American Great Lakes, where fish from polluted waters may form a relatively large part of the diet. Several investigators from Japan have measured the daily intake of PCBs in food; the highest mean value recorded was 48 μg/day, of which 90% was from fish (Kobayashi, 1972); the lowest was 8 μg/day (Ushio et al., 1974).

In much of Europe and North America, however, the daily intake of fish is in the region of 30–40 g and most of the fish is taken from waters of low pollution and contains PCB levels of not more than 0.1 mg/kg. Berglund (1972) has estimated that the daily intake of PCBs from fish in Sweden is in the region of 1 μg, though if the fish consumed were solely

Baltic herring, the intake would be about 10 µg. It is difficult to make an assessment of the PCB intake from foods other than fish. Westöö et al. (1971, 1972), in their extensive study of the Swedish diet, reported that most foods contained PCB levels of less than 0.1 mg/kg; it may be concluded that this corresponds to a daily intake of less than 100 µg. The conclusion that foods other than fish may make a greater contribution to the PCB content of the diet can be drawn from the survey in the USA reported by Kolbye (1972), and also from a Swiss study of three different types of home-prepared meals, not containing fish, which were found to contain 6, 41, and 84 µg of PCBs, respectively (Zimmerli & Marek, 1973).

The figures for the PCB content of human milk (section 5.5.5.3) indicate that most nursing mothers excreted about 30 µg/day by this route, and in some areas up to 100 µg/day. It may be assumed that only a portion of the PCBs absorbed was excreted by this route, so that the daily intake could have been more than 100 µg.

It may be concluded that, in the more industrialized countries, the average daily PCB intake from the diet has rarely been less than 5 µg or greater than 100 µg; it is likely that the non-dietary sources of exposure detailed in section 5.5.4 have made a significant contribution, but this cannot be estimated at this time. In any area, the intake depends not only on the diet, but also on social domestic and environmental conditions; the influence of these factors on the daily intake cannot readily be quantified.

6. METABOLISM

6.1 Absorption

The experiments of Vos & Beems (1971) who applied several commercial PCBs to rabbit skin and found systemic effects (see section 7.1.1.4) indicate that PCBs can penetrate the skin. Early cases of human poisoning from occupational exposure were probably due to a combination of skin absorption and inhalation. Experimental studies on rats by Benthe et al. (1972a) showed that an aerosol containing Aroclor 1242 (particle size 0.5–3.0 µm) was readily absorbed through the lungs.

Although one means of entry of PCBs into aquatic food chains is through the consumption of plankton by fish, aquatic organisms can also absorb PCBs in solution in the ambient water, presumably mainly through the gills (see section 4.3). Salmon eggs can also absorb PCBs from water (Johansson et al., 1970), and Södergren & Svensson 1973 concluded that mayfly nymphs could take in PCBs from water through the gills and the integument.

Recent work with chlorobiphenyl isomers administered orally to rodents at levels up 100 mg/kg of body weight for lower chlorinated compounds and up to 5 mg/kg for the higher chlorinated compounds, showed that 90% of the compounds were rapidly absorbed (Albro & Fishbein, 1972; Berlin et al., 1973; Melvås & Brandt, 1973). Cholestyramine, a basic anion exchange resin, was shown to interfere with intestinal absorption of KC-400 in mice (Tanaka & Araki, 1974).

PCTs have been shown to be absorbed from the gut (Sosa-Lucero et al., 1973) but very little information is available on the rate of absorption.

6.2   Tissue Distribution of PCBs

Grant et al. (1971a) demonstrated that 4 days after an oral dose of Aroclor 1254 at 500 mg/kg was given to rats, the concentrations of PCBs in fat, liver, and brain were 996, 116, and 40 mg/kg, respectively. Similar results showing that the highest concentration was in fat, were obtained in rats given Aroclor 1254 in the diet (Curley et al., 1971), in boars (Platonow et al., 1972), cows (Platonow & Chen, 1973), and in pigeons and quail (Bailey & Bunyan, 1972). In the experiments of Curley

Table 6. Tissue distribution of PCBs (mg/kg wet weight) in rats fed Aroclor 1254 (Grant et al., 1974), Aroclor 1242, or Aroclor 1016 (Burse et al., 1974) at 100 mg/kg for about 6 months

| Tissue | PCB levels in tissue (mg/kg) | | |
	Aroclor 1254	Aroclor 1242	Aroclor 1016
Blood	0.40	0.53 (plasma)	0.38 (plasma)
Liver	16	4.21	7.86
Brain	3.4	1,69	2.98
Kidneys	—	1.89	3.21
Heart	7.3	—	—
Fat	32.0	110	236
Urine	—	0.03	0.28

et al. (1971), the tissue concentrations initially showed a rapid rise and thereafter a slow increase while the PCB diet was being administered; Grant et al. (1974) fed diets containing Aroclor 1254 at 0.2, 20, and 100 mg/kg to rats for 8 months, during which period the tissue concentrations reached a steady state that was dose-dependent (Table 6). Similar tissue distribution data for Aroclors 1016 and 1242 have been reported by Burse et al. (1974) and for Kanechlor-400 by Yoshimura et al. (1971).

PCB deposition, in general, depends on the fat content of the tissue (section 5.4.2). Residues in trout, receiving Aroclor 1254 in doses of 15 mg/kg in the diet, stabilized after 16 weeks while the absolute quantity continued to increase as the fish grew (Lieb et al., 1974).

More detailed information on the tissue distribution of PCBs and their metabolites has been obtained by the administration of pure ^{14}C-labelled compounds, using both whole-body autoradiography and scintillation counting of tissue samples. Berlin et al. (1975) demonstrated that after a single oral dose of ^{14}C-labelled 2,5,2',4',5'-pentachlorobiphenyl, radioactivity rapidly entered the circulation of mice and was distributed in the tissues, particularly in the liver, kidneys, lungs, and adrenals. Subsequently, the radioactivity in the body fat increased, rising to a maximum within 4–24 h. In most other tissues the radioactivity decreased rapidly after dosing, but the authors noted a special affinity for the skin, the bronchiolar epithelium of the lungs, and certain glandular secreting tissue. Soon after administration of the dose, radioactivity appeared in bile and was excreted in the faeces. Similar results were obtained by Melvås & Brandt (1973) with 2,4,2',4'-tetrachlorobiphenyl in the mouse, and with 2,4,2',3'- and 2,4,3',4'-tetrachlorobiphenyls in the quail; in the mouse they found a high affinity for the adrenal cortex, the corpora lutea, and glandular secreting tissue, and in the quail the radioactivity in egg yolk was high, exceeding that in fat. Brandt & Ullberg (unpublished report 1973) found a similar pattern after administration of hexa- and octachlorobiphenyls to mice.

6.3   Tissue Distribution of PCTs

Diets containing Aroclor 5460 at levels of 10, 100, and 1000 mg/kg were administered to rats for 7 days (Sosa-Lucero et al., 1973). Table 7 shows the tissue distribution obtained in this study in rats fed with

Table 7. Tissue distribution (mg/kg wet weight) of PCTs (Aroclor 5460) in rats fed dietary levels of 100 mg/kg for 7 days (Sosa-Lucero et al., 1973) and fed PCB (Aroclor 1254) at 100 mg/kg for 9 days (Curley et al., 1971)

Tissue	Aroclor 5460	Aroclor 1254
Blood	1.32	0.1
Liver	47	6
Brain	5.1	4
Kidneys	15.1	5
Heart	21.5	—
Fat	—	180

Aroclor 5460 at 100 mg/kg body weight and the values in rats fed with Aroclor 1254 at 100 mg/kg body weight in a similar study (Curley et al., 1971). After oral administration of Aroclor 5460 to the cod, the concentration of PCTs in the liver was more than 100 times that in muscle on a wet weight basis (Addison et al., 1972), a ratio found by Jensen et al. (1973) for PCBs in the cod.

6.4   Placental Transport

Aroclors 1221 and 1254 were found to cross the placenta of rabbits, when administered orally to does during gestation. The concentration in fetal tissues was dose-dependent and much less with Aroclor 1221 than with Aroclor 1254; with the latter, the concentration in the fetal liver was greater than that in the maternal liver (Grant et al., 1971b). Curley et al. (1973a) found some placental transport of Aroclor 1254 in the rat. Platonow & Chen (1973) demonstrated that the PCBs in the fetal kidney of a cow dosed with Aroclor 1254 was greater than that in the mother. Placental transfer of polychlorinated biphenyls has also been reported in the mouse (Berlin et al., 1975; Melvås & Brandt, 1973; Brandt & Ullberg, unpublished report 1973).

PCB concentration in human umbilical blood has been shown to be about 25% of that in maternal blood (Taki et al., 1973). Placental transfer of PCBs was observed in Yusho patients (Tsukamoto et al., 1969).

No information is available on the placental transfer of PCTs.

6.5   Excretion and Elimination

6.5.1   Milk

Saschenbrecker et al. (1972) found that after oral administration of doses of Aroclor 1254 of   10, and 100 mg/kg in diet to cows, 6.27 and 74.5 mg/litre, respectively, appeared in the milk after 24 hours. These levels were reduced to less than one-half within 3 days but traces remained at 50 days. Cows receiving 200 mg of Aroclor 1254 daily reached a steady state concentration of 61 mg/kg in milk fat and 42 mg/kg in body fat after 10 days (Fries et al., 1973). The PCBs in milk survived processing into dairy products, and most was located in milk fat (Platonow et al., 1971). PCBs have also been found in human milk (see section 5.5.5.3).

6.5.2   Eggs

Several investigations have demonstrated the presence of high levels of PCBs in the eggs of seabirds (Risebrough & de Lappe, 1972). An incident has been reported in which PCB contamination of poultry food was toxic to chickens and decreased the hatchability of eggs which also contained PCB residues (Pichirallo, 1971). In a laboratory study, Scott et al. (1975) fed Aroclor 1248 to chickens at dietary concentrations of 0, 0.5, 1.0, 10, and 20 mg/kg. After 8 weeks, the approximate PCB levels in eggs were 0, 0.22, 0.41, 3.1 and 7.0 mg/kg respectively. Jensen & Sundström (1974) found 33% of an oral dose of 2,4,5,2',4',5'-hexachlorobiphenyl administered to quails was excreted in eggs over a period of 10 days; eggs also provided a major route of excretion in the pheasant (Dahlgren et al., 1971).

6.5.3 Urine and faeces

All investigators agree that only traces of PCBs can be found in the urine of dosed animals, and that faeces provide a major route of elimination. When the analysis of faeces is limited to the determination of unchanged PCBs, the recovery of the dose administered is incomplete; in boars receiving single or repeated doses of Aroclor 1254, not more than 16% of the dose was recovered from the faeces and less than 1% in urine (Platonow et al., 1972). Better recoveries have been obtained with PCB labelled with radioactive isotopes. Yoshimura et al. (1971) found 70% of the activity from a dose of tritium-labelled Kanechlor 400 in faeces and 2% in urine over a 4-week period. Berlin et al. (1974, 1975) found over 75% of the activity from ^{14}C-labelled penta- and hexachlorobiphenyls in faeces and less than 2% in urine; most of the faecal excretion consisted of PCB metabolites (see section 6.6.1). Similar results were obtained by Melvås & Brandt (1973) with tetrachlorobiphenyls.

6.6 Biotransformation

6.6.1 Metabolic degradation

Most investigators studying the tissue distribution of PCBs after administration of commercial mixtures have noted a relative reduction of the gas–liquid chromatographic peaks with shorter retention times, corresponding to the lower chlorinated biphenyls. This has been reported in the rat (Grant et al., 1971a; Curley et al., 1971), the rabbit (Grant et al., 1971b), the cow (Platanow & Chen, 1973), and in pigeons and quails (Koeman et al., 1969; Bailey & Bunyan, 1972). Samples of tissues from animals and man (see table 3, pp. 20–21) that have absorbed PCBs from the environment have shown, on analysis, a pattern of peaks approaching that of PCB mixtures with more than 50% chlorination, although the major manufactured products contain 42% of chlorine or less. This has led to the belief that the rate of metabolic attack on PCBs decreases with increasing chlorination. Studies on single PCBs with 1, 2, 4, or 5 chlorine atoms have shown that these are more readily excreted as metabolites in faeces by mammals and birds and remain for a shorter time in fatty tissues than most PCBs with 6 or more chlorine atoms (Berlin et al., 1975; Hutzinger et al., 1972a; Melvås & Brandt, 1973; Brandt & Ullberg, unpublished report 1973). See also section 6.6.2.

The administration to rats of diets containing Aroclors 1016 or 1242 at a concentration of 100 mg/kg resulted in a steady state in adipose tissue for both compounds in about 4 months. When gas chromatographic traces were compared with those for standard PCB mixtures a difference in the gas–liquid chromatographic pattern, that is disappearance of the peaks with short retention times was noted. After exposure to PCBs was discontinued, a major portion of the PCBs was eliminated from the body in 4 months. However, 20% of the total PCBs in Aroclor 1242 with longer retention times were present after 6 months, and 10% of the total PCBs of Aroclor 1016 with longer retention times were present in adipose tissue after 5 months. (Burse et al., 1974).

The excretion of monohydroxy metabolites of 3,4,3',4'-tetrachloro-biphenyl and 2,4,3',4'-tetrachlorobiphenyl (orally administered) in rats has been demonstrated by Yoshimura & Yamamoto (1973). Yoshimura et al. (1973), Yamamoto & Yoshimura (1973), Yoshimura & Yamamoto (1974), and Yoshimura et al. (1974). They demonstrated that the metabolites of the first isomer were 2-hydroxy or 5-hydroxy compounds while the metabolites of the second isomer were 5-hydroxy and 3-hydroxy compounds. All hydroxy metabolites were excreted non-conjugated via the bile and no parent isomers were found in the bile. Yoshimura & Yamamoto (1975) found that unchanged 2,4,3',4'-tetrachlorobiphenyl was excreted through the intestine, when it was intravenously injected in rats with the bile duct ligated, while no metabolite of this isomer was excreted by this route.

Hutzinger et al. (1972a) demonstrated the presence of hydroxylated derivatives of mono-, di-, and tetrachlorobiphenyls in the excreta of rats and pigeons but not of trout and were unable to detect hydroxylated 2,4,5,2',4',5'-hexachlorobiphenyl. Berlin et al. (1975) isolated a hydroxy derivative of 2,5,2',4',5'-pentachlorobiphenyl from mouse faeces, and Jensen & Sundström (1975) have shown that although 2,4,5,2',4',5'-hexachlorobiphenyl is excreted very slowly, a hydroxy derivative could be detected in rat faeces. Hutzinger et al. (1974), however, showed that this compound was also dechlorinated by the rabbit and excreted as the hydroxy derivative of pentachlorobiphenyl. Gardner et al. (1973) detected hydroxylated metabolites in the urine of rabbits dosed with 2,5,2′,5′-tetrachlorobiphenyl together with a dihydroxy derivative which they regarded as evidence for the formation of an arene oxide (epoxide) intermediate (see section 6.5.3). Jansson et al. (1975) have identified up to 26 mono- and dihydroxylated metabolites of PCB in the bile and faeces of wild grey seal and guillemot from the Baltic.

There is little information on the biotransformation of PCTs. Addison et al. (1972), using gas–liquid chromatography, noted a loss of PCTs with a shorter retention time in the excreta of a cod dosed orally with Aroclor 5460; the same loss was observed in rat faeces after the administration of a diet containing Aroclor 5460 (Sosa-Lucero et al., 1973).

6.6.2 The effect of structure on retention

While each of the components of mixtures of PCBs has a different pattern of retention and elimination in different species, the measurement of biological half-times for PCB mixtures in tissues has provided useful information. Bailey & Bunyan (1972) found the half-time of PCBs in the fat of quail and pigeon, after cessation of dosing with Aroclor 1242, or with Aroclor 1254, to be 50 days and 125 days, respectively. A half-time of about 200 days was recorded in the fat of rats after feeding with Aroclor 1254 (Grant et al., 1974). Berlin et al. (1975) noted that in mice dosed with a pentachlorobiphenyl there was an initial fairly rapid elimination while the PCB level in the liver was high, followed by a slower elimination when most of the PCB was located in fat. It seems likely that the mobilization of PCBs from fat, and therefore their half-time in the body, depends upon their rates of metabolism. Berlin et al. (1974) investigated the hypothesis that the ability of a PCB to be readily degraded with a half-time of a few days depended upon the presence of two adjacent unsubstituted carbon atoms in the molecule rather than on the number of chlorine atoms, although the presence of such unsubstituted pairs depends to a large extent on the degree of chlorination. They came to the conclusion that this hypothesis probably applied to unsubstituted pairs in the 3,4-position, but that in the 2,3-position, their susceptibility to metabolic degradation was much influenced by the presence of chlorines in the o-position of the ring bridge.

Jensen & Sundström (1974) demonstrated that the retention of PCBs in human fat is also influenced by o-chlorine substitution (Table 3, pp. 20–21).

7. EXPERIMENTAL STUDIES ON THE EFFECTS OF PCBs AND PCTs

7.1 Toxic Effects in Different Species

Most of the available information on the toxicity of the PCBs has been obtained from studies on commercial mixtures. The much smaller amount of information available concerning the impurities in commercial products and PCTs, is given in sections 7.2 and 7.3.

7.1.1 Mammals

7.1.1.1 *Acute oral and intravenous toxicity*

Earlier work by the Monsanto Company indicated a low acute oral toxicity for the Aroclors, the LD_{50}s to rats ranging from 4.0 g/kg for Aroclor 1221 to 11.3 g/kg for Aroclor 1262 (Panel on Hazardous Trace Substances, 1972). More recent work has demonstrated a slightly higher toxicity (Bruckner et al., 1973; Grant & Philips, 1974). With a single intravenous dose the LD_{50} for Aroclor 1254 was 358 mg/kg body weight in adult female Sherman rats (Linder et al., 1974). The acute oral LD_{50} for Aroclor 1254 in the same strain and sex was between 4 and 10 g/kg (Kimbrough et al., 1972). According to Bruckner et al. (1973), severely poisoned animals showed weight loss, ataxia, diarrhoea, and chromo-dacryorrhoea, and they considered progressive dehydration and central nervous depression were the causes of death. In rats, vacuolation in the liver and kidneys was observed (Bruckner et al., 1973) and also ulceration of the gastric and duodenal mucosa (Kimbrough et al., 1972).

Yamamoto & Yoshimura (1973) found the intraperitoneal LD_{50} of 2,4,3',4'-tetrachlorobiphenyl in mice to be 2.15 g/kg body weight and that of the 5-hydroxy derivative, which is the main *in vivo* metabolite, to be 0.43 g/kg body weight.

7.1.1.2 *Subacute oral toxicity*

After repeated administration, the PCBs have a cumulative toxic action. In a group of rats receiving Aroclor 1254 at a dose of 1 g/kg of diet, deaths occurred between the 28th and 53rd days of feeding (Tucker & Crabtree, 1970), and with Phenochlor DP6 at 2 g/kg of diet, deaths occurred between the 12th and 26th days (Vos & Koeman, 1970). In the latter experiment enlarged livers, small spleens, and a progressive chemically-induced hepatic porphyria were seen at autopsy. Repeated weekly oral administration of 150 mg of Aroclors 1221, 1242 or 1254 to rabbits for

14 weeks produced liver enlargement and damage with Aroclor 1242 and no effect with Aroclor 1221 (Koller & Zinkl, 1973). Allen et al. (1974) administered diets containing Aroclor 1248 at the concentration of 25 mg/kg of diet to 6 female rhesus monkeys for two months; facial oedema, loss of hair, and acne developed after 1 month and one animal died with severe gastritis 2 months after removal from experimental diet. PCB concentrations in the body fat of the animals, after two months of treatment, averaged 127 mg/kg while 8 months later the value declined to 34 mg/kg.

Mink appear to be unusually sensitive to PCBs. Aulerich et al. (1973) administered diets containing PCB levels of 30 mg/kg (10 mg/kg each of Aroclors 1242, 1248, and 1254) to adult mink and demonstrated 100% mortality within 6 months. PCB residues in the brains of these mink averaged about 11 mg/kg and were approximately twice the level observed in other tissues. Four months of feeding Aroclor 1254 at levels of 5 and 10 mg/kg demonstrated a dose-dependent retardation of weight gain of growing female mink. Female mink fed a diet supplemented with Aroclor 1254 at 5 mg/kg for 9 months failed to produce offspring (Ringer et al., 1972).

7.1.1.3 *Chronic oral toxicity*

Aroclors 1242, 1254, and 1260 have been administered for 18 months to rats at 1, 10 and 100 mg/kg in the diet (Keplinger et al., 1971). No adverse effects were recorded with the three Aroclors at 10 mg/kg but with Aroclors 1242 and 1254 at 100 mg/kg there was an increase in liver weight and a reduced survival of litters. In similar experiments on dogs, there was a reduced weight gain with Aroclors 1254 and 1260 in the diet at a level of 100 mg/kg (Keplinger et al., 1971). In the experiments reported by Kimbrough et al. (1972), male rats survived Aroclor 1260 in the diet at 1 g/kg (71.4 mg/kg body weight) for 8 months but 8/10 females died at this dose, 2/10 died at 500 mg/kg, and 1/10 at 100 mg/kg (7.2 mg/kg body weight). With Aroclors 1254 and 1260, a dose-dependent increase in liver weight in male rats was significant down to 20 mg/kg (1.4 mg/kg body weight) in the diet; with females the liver enlargement occurred only at diet levels of 500 mg/kg and higher. The livers showed an orange fluorescence, the cells were enlarged and vacuolated with lipid inclusions; there was also much increased smooth endoplasmic reticulum, and what was termed "adenofibrosis" was present, being more marked with Aroclor 1254 (see section 7.8). Grant et al. (1974) fed diets containing Aroclor 1254 at 0, 2, 20, and 100 mg/kg to rats for 246 days followed by 180 days on a PCB-free diet; after 246 days the body weight of the 100 mg/kg rats was significantly less than that of the controls and the liver weight was greater. The most notable change in the livers on histological examination was the appearance of fat microdroplets in the centrilobular region; this effect was dose-dependent and not seen in the rats receiving the 2 mg/kg diet and was reversible when the rats were returned to a normal diet.

Liver enlargement has been described by a number of authors, in a number of species, with different PCB mixtures and pure isomers and it is considered to be due primarily to hypertrophy of the smooth endoplasmic reticulum of the liver cells (Vos & Beems, 1971; Allen et al., 1973; Kimbrough, 1974; Nishizumi, 1970) but with large enough doses (oral intubation of about 150 mg/kg body weight/week for 14 weeks) of Aroclor 1254 and 1242, it progressed to frank liver damage (Koller & Zinkl, 1973). The smooth endoplasmic reticulum may condense in the liver cell and form hyalin inclusions and this may be accompanied by a loss of enzyme activity. Lipid accumulation, pigment deposition, nuclear changes, and necrosis may also occur (Vos & Notenboom-Ram, 1972).

The rhesus monkey is the only species reported to show signs of poisoning similar to those in human Yusho patients (see section 8). The administration of Aroclor 1248 at 2.5 and 5.0 mg/kg of diet for 1 year produced periorbital oedema, alopecia, erythema, and acneiform lesions involving the face and neck within 1–2 months. The effects were less marked in male monkeys. At 25 mg/kg of diet, one out of a group of six died, and at 100 and 300 mg/kg the mortality approached 100% within 2–3 months. Animals more severely affected showed hypertrophic hyperplastic gastritis with ulceration, anaemia, hyperproteinaemia and bone marrow hypoplasia. The survivors still showed signs of poisoning 8 months after exposure (Allen & Norback, 1973; Allen et al., 1974; Allen 1975).

7.1.1.4   *Dermal toxicity*

Vos & Beems (1971) have confirmed earlier reports that PCBs damage the follicular epithelium in experimental animals. They applied three commercial 60% chlorinated mixtures, Clophen A60, Phenochlor DP6, and Aroclor 1260 to rabbit skin at a daily dose of 118 mg/50 cm^2 (5 times per week) for 38 days. After initial reddening, transverse wrinkling developed with hyperplasia and hyperkeratosis of the epidermal and follicular epithelium. These effects were more marked with Clophen and Phenochlor than with the Aroclor.

During these experiments, deaths occurred in the Clophen- and Phenochlor-treated groups but not in the Aroclor group. Kidney lesions were seen in all groups; liver damage was least in the Aroclor group. There was atrophy of the thymus cortex and a reduction of germinal centres of the lymph nodes as well as lymphopenia, and some animals in all groups showed oedema of the abdominal and thoracic cavities, subcutaneous tissue, and pericardium. Faecal excretion of copro- and protoporphyrins was increased by all three PCBs but was lowest with Aroclor 1260. Vos & Beems attributed the greater severity of the effects observed with Clophen and Phenochlor to the presence of toxic impurities (see section 7.2). In another comparative dermal toxicity study in rabbits (Vos & Notenboom-Ram, 1972), skin lesions in Aroclor 1260-treated animals were more severe than in animals treated with 2,4,5,2′,4′,5′-hexachlorobiphenyl. In a Japanese study, no differences in skin lesions were observed in rabbits after dermal applications of Kanechlor 400, Kanechlor 500, or 3,4,3′,4′-tetrachlorobiphenyl (Komatsu & Kikuchi, 1972).

7.1.1.5 *Inhalation toxicity*

Only one inhalation study has been reported using Aroclor 1242 and 1254 (Treon et al., 1956). Rats, mice, rabbits, and guinea pigs were exposed to Aroclor 1242 or 1254 vapours for five days a week for several weeks at concentrations ranging from 1.5 to 8.6 mg/m^3. At these concentrations Aroclor 1254 produced liver enlargement in rats.

7.1.2 Birds

The acute oral toxicity of Aroclors 1242 and 1254 is low for the mallard duck, the LD_{50}s being greater than 2 g/kg body weight (Tucker & Crabtree, 1970). Published figures for the lethal dose for birds after repeated administration are very variable; it appears to be dependent on the species and age of the bird, the method of administration, the degree of chlorination of the PCBs, and the presence of impurities (Vos, 1972). Heath et al. (1970) determined the dietary concentrations of Aroclors 1232 to 1262, administered over a 5-day period, that were required to kill 50% of groups of mallards, pheasants, and quails. The concentrations were in the range of 500 to over 5000 mg/kg, with the bobwhite quail the most sensitive and the Japanese quail the least. There was a positive relationship between the percentage of chlorine in a technical Aroclor and its toxicity. The relationship held true for those containing less than 60% chlorine, Aroclor 1260 and 1262 deviating slightly. Mallards were relatively less responsive to chlorine content than the three gallinaceous species. Prestt et al. (1970) found a 50% mortality in Bengalese finches receiving a daily oral dose of Aroclor 1254 at 254 mg/kg body weight for 56 days; cormorants have been killed with a cumulative dose of 5.7 g of Clophen A60, but herons were more resistant (Koeman et al., 1973).

The toxicity to chickens of diets containing Phenochlor DP6, Clophen A60, or Aroclor 1260 at 400 mg/kg has been studied by Vos & Koeman

(1970). The first two produced a 100% mortality with survival times of 24.3 and 20.5 days, but there was only 15% mortality with the Aroclor over the 60-day test period. The authors demonstrated the presence of impurities in the Phenochlor and Clophen (Vos et al., 1970). The results of Flick et al. (1965) and Platonow & Funnel (1971) indicate that chickens can survive 200 mg/kg in the diet for several months, but that deaths may occur at 250 mg/kg, though Rehfeld et al. (1971) found a much higher toxicity, recording 1/30 deaths with Aroclor 1248 at 30 mg/kg of diet over 25 days and 16/30 at 50 mg/kg. Keplinger et al. (1971) found decreased growth in chickens receiving Aroclor 1242 at 10 mg/kg and Aroclor 1254 at 100 mg/kg of diet, but no effects with Aroclor 1260 at 100 mg/kg. Birds severely poisoned with PCBs show tremors, ataxia, and ruffling and loss of feathers. Oedema of the abdominal and peritoneal cavities has been a characteristic sign at autopsy in some experiments (Flick et al., 1965) and this was observed in a very large number of chickens killed in Japan by the contamination of their feed with Kanechlor KC400 (Kohanawa et al., 1969a, 1969b). Enlargement of the kidneys and sometimes of the liver has been reported; some authors have noted a reduction in the size of the spleen, comb, and testes, an enlargement of the adrenals and thyroid, and a pale pancreas. No pathological signs were observed by Dahlgren et al. (1972) that could account for the deaths of pheasants, which occurred with a cumulative intake of about 900 mg of Aroclor 1254 (daily oral administration of 20 or 200 mg to 11-week-old hens); they found a mean concentration of 520 mg/kg in brain tissue at death and it is possible that effects in the central nervous system were a contributory cause.

7.1.3 Aquatic organisms

7.1.3.1 *Fish*

Stalling & Mayer (1972) report an oral LD_{50} of more than 1.5 g/kg for rainbow trout with Aroclors 1242 and 1260. A 15 mg/kg oral dose to cod affected their ability to maintain an upright position in rotating water (Lindahl, unpublished report 1974).

The assessment of toxicity to fish by adding PCBs to aquarium water is subject to considerable error on account of the different solubilities of the components. Zitko (1970) claims the aqueous solubility of Aroclor 1221 to be 3.8–5 mg/litre and that of Aroclor 1254 to be 0.3–0.5 mg/litre. Stalling & Mayer (1972) report the 96-hour LC_{50}s on the cut-throat trout to be 1.17 mg/litre for Aroclor 1221 and up to 60 mg/litre for Aroclor 1260, where the solubility is clearly exceeded. In the more prolonged experiments of these authors (Table 8), most of the concentrations are

Table 8. Intermittent-flow bioassays of Aroclors against three species of fish[a]

| Aroclor | Species | LC$_{50}$(µg/litre) | | | | | |
		5 days	10 days	15 days	20 days	25 days	30 days
1254	Rainbow trout	156	8	—	—	—	—
1260		—	240	94	21	—	—
DDT		2.26	0.87	0.26	—	—	—
1242	Bluegills	154	72	54	—	—	—
1248		307	160	76	10	—	—
1254		—	443	204	135	54	—
1260		—	—	—	245	212	151
1242	Channel catfish	—	174	107	—	—	—
1248		—	225	127	—	—	—
1254		—	—	741	300	113	—
1260		—	—	—	296	166	137
1248[b]	Bluegills	137	76	—	—	—	—
1248[c]	Channel catfish	—	94	57	—	—	—

[a] From Stalling & Mayer (1972).

[b] Temperature, 20°C; alkalinity 260 mg/litre pH 7.4.

[c] Temperature, 27°C.

within the solubility limits and therefore more reliable. In more prolonged experiments, Hansen et al. (1971) found deaths in fish exposed for up to 45 days to Aroclor 1254 at 5 µg/litre, but none at 1 µg/litre. These results show that the effect of PCBs is cumulative in fish and that the toxicity decreases with increasing chlorination.

Young fish appear to be more sensitive to PCBs than adults, 96-hour LC$_{50}$s for newly hatched fathead minnows were 15 and 8 µg/litre, respectively for Aroclors 1242 and 1254. Growth of young fathead minnows and flagfish was affected above 2.2 µg/litre (Nebeker et al., 1974). There is no information on pathological changes in fish that might be related to the lethal action of PCBs; Hansen et al. (1971) found that fish survived exposure to Aroclor 1254 at 5 µg/litre, but died later, after being returned to clean water, with signs of a lowered resistance to infection. Pathological changes were observed in kidney, spleen, and liver of rainbow trout fed Aroclor 1254 at 10 or 100 mg/kg of diet for up to 330 days (Nestel & Budd, 1975).

7.1.3.2 Aquatic invertebrates

The results of several investigations into the toxicity of PCBs to aquatic invertebrates have been reported by Stalling & Mayer (1972). The exposure of a variety of scud (*Gammarus pseudolimnaeus*) to PCBs showed a decreased toxicity with increasing chlorination; 4-day LC$_{50}$s of 10, 52, and 2400 µg/litre were obtained with Aroclors 1242, 1248 and 1254, respectively. The threshold for survival, growth, and reproduction of

Gammarus pseudolimnaeus exposed to Aroclor 1248 was about 5 µg/litre and was the same for *Daphnia magna*. With the crayfish, 7-day LC_{50}s were 30 µg/litre (Aroclor 1242) and 80 µg/litre (Aroclor 1254) and with the glass shrimp, 3 µg/litre (Aroclor 1254). Wildish (1970) found that mortality in *Gammarus oceanicus* was dependent on the duration of exposure to Aroclor 1254 at levels above 10 µg/litre. Stalling & Mayer (1972) reported the 15-day LC_{50} of Aroclor 1254 for immature pink shrimp to be 0.94 µg/litre.

7.1.3.3 *Microorganisms*

The growth of certain marine diatoms is inhibited by Aroclor 1254 at 10–25 µg/litre, but marine and freshwater algae are more resistant, being unaffected by 100 µg/litre (Mosser et al., 1972). Fisher et al. (1972) found that phytoplankton from the Sargasso Sea did not grow in Aroclor 1254 at 10 µg/litre, though phytoplankton from estuarine and coastal waters were not much affected by this concentration. Keil et al. (1971) report that the growth of a diatom was inhibited by Aroclor 1242 at 100 µg/litre with a reduction of RNA synthesis, but that 10 µg/litre had no effect.

The growth of cultures of lake bacteria was not inhibited by concentrations of Aroclors 1221, 1242, and 1254 in excess of solubility, and Aroclors 1221 and 1242 could be utilized as the sole source of carbon and energy (Wong & Kaiser, 1975).

7.2   Toxicity of Impurities in Commercial PCBs

Vos & Koeman (1970) observed that Phenochlor DP6 and Clophen A60 were more toxic to chickens than was Aroclor 1260 (see section 7.1.2) and Vos & Beems (1971) showed a similar difference in the dermal toxicity to the rabbit (see section 7.1.1.4). Vos et al. (1970) subdivided Clophen A60 and Phenochlor DP6 into non-polar PCBs and polar fractions and found polar components that were not detectable in a similar fraction from Aroclor 1260. Phenoclor DP6, Clophen A60, and the polar fraction from Clophen A60 produced a high mortality in the chick embryo test but the polar fraction from Aroclor 1260 did not. A difference between the three fractions was seen in the development of skin lesions in the rabbit (Vos & Beems, 1971). Mass spectrographic analysis indicated that the impurities were tetra- and pentachlorodibenzofurans. Additional contaminants were chlorinated naphthalenes. Vos et al. (1970) calculated that the maximum level of chlorinated dibenzofurans in Clophen A60 was 5 mg/kg and in Phenochlor DP6, 20 mg/kg. They calculated that the chlorinated dibenzofurans were approximately one order of magnitude less toxic than the chlorinated benzodioxins, and considered that they were mainly responsible for the toxicity of the polar fraction and for the difference in toxicity between the three commercial PCB mixtures.

Recently, chlorinated dibenzofurans were detected in the PCB-contaminated oil that was responsible for the Yusho disease in Japan (see section 8, p. 65).

In 1961, Bauer et al. demonstrated the toxicity of a mixture of tri- and tetrachlorodibenzofurans; a single oral dose of 0.5–1.0 mg/kg body weight caused severe and often lethal liver necrosis in rabbits. Application to the rabbit ear resulted in hyperplasia and hyperkeratosis. Similar toxic effects were found with 2,3,7,8-tetrachlorodibenzo-p-dioxin in doses that were 10 times lower than those found to be toxic in the case of chlorinated dibenzofurans. See also the review by Kimbrough (1974). 2,3,7,8-Tetrachlorodibenzofuran, which has recently been shown to be present in PCBs (Bowes et al., 1975) caused mortality in chickens after 8–15 days when they were dosed orally with 5 µg/kg/day. A single oral dose of 4000 µg/kg was not lethal to mice. Porphyria was not observed in chicks or mice (Goldstein et al., 1975a). In comparison, 8 out of 10 chicks died after 9–19 days when dosed orally with 2,3,7,8-tetrachlorodibenzo-p-dioxin at 1 µg/kg body weight/day (Schwetz et al., 1973). The oral LD_{50} of 2,3,7,8-tetrachlorodibenzofuran in guinea pigs is approximately 7 µg/kg body weight, which is less than one order of magnitude higher than that of 2,3,7,8-tetrachlorodibenzo-p-dioxin (Moore, 1975).

Using low resolution mass spectrometry, McKinney (1975) found metabolites in the excreta of chickens fed 2,4,6,2′,4′,6′-hexachlorobiphenyl which had correct masses for chlorodibenzofurans. In addition, by perchlorination, he identified octachlorodibenzofuran again by low resolution mass spectrometry. The 2,4,6,2′,4′,6′-hexachlorobiphenyl isomer is not found in commercial mixtures.

Zitko et al. (1972b) looked for the presence of chlorinated dibenzo-furans in fish and fish products taken from a contaminated coastal area. The samples included shark tissues, cormorant and herring gull eggs, herring oil, and herring fishmeal. The detection limit of the method was 0.01–0.02 mg/kg in the sample. No chlorinated dibenzofurans were detected, although the authors admit that the limit of detection was not sufficiently low to detect amounts that might exert a significant toxic action. Curley et al. (1975) detected a component which had a 4 Cl isotopic cluster and a mass number of 304 corresponding with that of tetrachloro-dibenzofuran in the urine of rats dosed with PCBs, but a positive identification was not made.

7.3   Toxicity of the PCTs

There have not been any systematic studies on the toxicity of the PCTs. Sosa-Lucero et al. (1973) administered diets containing Aroclor 5460 at 0, 10, 100, and 1000 mg/kg to groups of rats for seven days. There were no adverse effects on health or body weight; a significant liver enlargement was recorded at the 1000 mg/kg level. In a test for estrogenic activity involving the stimulation of glycogen response in the immature rat uterus, Aroclor 5460 was inactive, as was Aroclor 1260 but Aroclor 5442 was more active than Arochlor 1242 (Bitman et al., 1972). A dietary level of Aroclor 5460 of 5000 mg/kg for 12 weeks caused decreased body weight and increased liver weight in rhesus monkeys (Allen & Norback, 1973); after 6 weeks, facial oedema, hair loss, and eye discharge were observed as described by the same authors in experiments with Aroclor 1248 (section 7.1.1.2), and similar gastric changes were also reported.

7.4   Biochemical Effects

7.4.1   Induction of enzymes

Several investigators have observed an increase in the smooth endoplasmic reticulum of liver cells after administration of PCBs (see section 7.1.1.3). This is accompanied by an induction of microsomal mixed function oxidase. Induction of microsomal enzyme activity is, like liver enlargement, more marked with the higher chlorinated PCBs and relatively low with Aroclors 1221 and 1016 (Villeneuve et al., 1971a, 1972; Bickers et al., 1972; Ecobichon & Comeau, 1974). The effect has also been demonstrated with single pure PCBs administered orally (Fujita et al., 1971); more recently this work has been confirmed by Johnstone et al. (1974) whose results are summarized in Table 9 and show a greater degree of enzyme induction with the higher chlorinated compounds.

Grant et al. (1974) found an increase in microsomal enzyme activity in rats receiving Aroclor 1254 at 20 mg/kg of diet for 246 days, but none at 2 mg/kg. Iverson et al. (1975) and Goldstein et al. (1975) compared the microsomal enzyme inducing potential of Aroclors 1242 and 1016. Iverson et al. (1975) found increased hepatic microsomal enzyme activity with both Aroclors in male rats receiving 21 daily oral doses of 1 mg/kg body weight, and with Aroclor 1242 in females at 10 mg/kg of body weight and with Aroclor 1016 at 100 mg/kg. PCBs administered to rats during pregnancy can induce microsomal enzyme activity in the placenta and fetus and this also occurs in the liver of newborn rats suckled by mothers

Table 9. Stimulation of microsomal enzyme activity by single chlorinated biphenyls

Chlorine substituents	Hepatic microsomal enzyme activity			
	O-demethylation	N-demethylation	aniline hydroxylation	nitro-reduction
4	0	0	0	0
2,2'	0	+	+	0
2,4'	0	0	+	0
4,4'	+ +	+ +	+ +	+
2,5,2',5'	0	+	+ +	+
2,4,2',4'	+ +	+ +	+ +	0
2,4,5,2',4',5'	+ +	+ +	+ +	+ +
2,3,5,2',3',5'	+ +	+ +	+	+ +
2,4,6,2',4',6'	+ +	+ +	+ +	+ +
2,3,4,5,2',3',4',5'	+ +	+ +	+ +	+ +

[a] After Johnstone et al. (1974).
  0   no activity.
  +   slight activity.
 + +   marked activity.

fed with diets containing PCBs (Alvares & Kappas, 1975). Benthe et al. (1972b) reported that when rats were stressed by food deprivation or cold, the PCB residues in adipose tissue were released during mobilization of the fat and caused increased hepatic microsomal enzyme activity.

7.4.2 Porphyria

Hepatic porphyria has been induced by a number of PCBs (Clophen A60, Phenoclor DP6, Aroclors 1016, 1242, 1254, and 1260) in the chicken, rabbit, Japanese quail, and the rat (Vos & Koeman 1970; Vos & Beems, 1971; Iverson et al., 1975; Vos et al., 1971; Goldstein et al., 1974, 1975a, 1975b). Porphyrin induction has been studied more extensively in rats. A dose-dependent increase in liver porphyrins has been observed in females receiving 21 daily oral doses of Aroclor 1242 at 10 and 100 mg/kg of body weight, but not at 1 mg/kg. Female rats were more sensitive than males, and Aroclor 1016 had less effect (Iverson et al., 1975). In rats receiving Aroclor 1254 at 100 mg/kg in the diet, the increase was usually delayed 2–4 months after the start of dosing (Goldstein, 1974) and was characterized by high hepatic and urinary levels of uroporphyrin. Disturbance of porphyrin biosynthesis had been connected with an increase of the rate limiting enzyme 2.3.1.37-δ-aminolaevulinate synthase (Vos et al., 1971; Goldstein 1974, 1975).

Kawanishi et al. (1973, 1974) have shown that the administration, in the diet, of Kanechlors KC-300 and KC-500 to rats at 500 mg/kg produced a marked increase in urinary excretion of copro- and uroporphyrins, and in faecal excretion of protoporphyrin, but no increase was observed with KC-400. Experimental administration of pure tetrachloro-biphenyls did not produce porphyria. However, porphyria did result from the repeated subcutaneous injection of KC-400 (total dose 1.8 g) to rabbits for 55 days (Miura et al., 1973).

7.4.3 Effects on steroid metabolism

PCBs have been shown to stimulate the activity of enzymes responsible for metabolizing steroids such as estrodiol and androsterone more effectively than does DDT or DDE (Risebrough et al., 1968; Lincer & Peakall, 1970). It has been suggested that effects on reproduction (see section 7.4) may be attributed to the induction of steroid-metabolizing enzymes (Kihlström et al., 1973). Long-term administration of daily oral doses of 0.025 mg Clophen A60 to 23 female NMRI strain mice caused a lengthening of the estrous cycle and a reduction in the frequency of implantation of ova (Örberg & Kihlström, 1973).

7.4.4 Other biochemical effects

Hepatic vitamin A has been reported by Villeneuve et al. (1971a) to be reduced to half the normal values in pregnant rabbits by Aroclor 1254. Similar observations have been made by Cecil et al. (1973) in male and female Japanese quails and in rats after feeding Aroclor 1242 at 100 mg/kg of diet. The 50% decrease in hepatic vitamin A found in male and female rats was also found in male and female quail provided that the latter were kept in the dark to prevent egg laying.

A lowering of hepatic vitamin A in rats, fed a 0.1% PCB diet (PCB not specified), was described by Innami et al. (1974). The rats given vitamin A supplement (3400 IU) plus PCB for 6 weeks showed better growth than those given PCB alone, while those given PCB and a vitamin A deficient diet showed significant growth retardation. On the PCB diet, the hepatic vitamin A level decreased to 20% of the normal level during the experimental period; supplementing the diet with 1000 IU did not re-establish the vitamin A level in the liver. Administration of 3000 IU of vitamin A with the PCB diet, however, allowed better than normal hepatic vitamin A levels to be re-established. The authors concluded that vitamin A may play a role in the detoxification of PCB rather than that PCB plays a role in the destructive metabolism of vitamin A.

Aroclor 1254 administered intraperitoneally to rats at 25 mg/kg body weight daily for 4 days caused a 4- to 5-fold increase in the biliary excretion of thyroxine during a 3-hour period. Biliary clearance was greatly elevated. Hypobilirubinaemia has been produced in rats by Bastomsky et al. (1975) who investigated the mechanism by administering daily intra-peritoneal injections of Aroclor 1254 (25 mg/kg body weight in corn oil) to female rats for 4 days, then measuring bilirubin glucuronide formation by hepatic microsomes *in vitro*. PCB treatment was not effective in increasing UDPglucuronosyltransferase (2.4.1.7) activity. Serum bilirubin levels were also significantly decreased by PCB treatment of Gunn rats, which are genetically deficient in UDPglucuronosyltransferase (2.4.1.7) activity.

7.4.5 Potentiation and antagonism by PCBs

As PCBs can stimulate microsomal enzyme activity, it is to be expected that they may potentiate the action of those chemicals that undergo microsomal activation, and decrease the action of those that are detoxified. Villeneuve et al. (1973) demonstrated the antagonistic effect by the reduction of phenobarbital sleeping time in rats receiving Aroclors 1242, 1254, and 1260 in their diet, but not in those receiving Aroclor 1221. Johnstone et al. (1974) have confirmed this with a series of single PCBs. Tanaka & Komatsu (1972) found that the hexobarbital-induced sleeping time in female rats was reduced to 49% of the control value by daily oral doses of Kanechlor 500 of 2 mg/kg for 3 days (total 6 mg/kg). When a daily dose of 0.4 mg/kg was given for 15 days (total 6 mg/kg), no reduction in sleeping time was observed. When this small dose was continued for 45 and 53 days, the reduction remained at 12–13%. Phillips et al. (1972) did not find any potentiation of the cholinesterase-inhibitory action of parathion in rats dosed with Aroclors 1221 and 1254; this does not necessarily imply that there was no enhanced activation of parathion, as a stimulation of detoxication may have occurred concurrently. A stimula-tion of parathion detoxication but not of activation has been demonstrated in rabbit microsomes (Villeneuve et al., 1971a). Lichtenstein (1972) reports a potentiation by PCBs of the toxicity of parathion to flies.

Cecil et al. (1975) have shown that the ability of PCTs to decrease phenobarbital sleeping time in quails is rather less than that of the PCBs.

Aroclor 1254 at 160 mg/kg of diet fed to 5-week old male and female Fischer-344 rats for 8 weeks reduced mortality due to feeding hexachloro-phene at a concentration of 600 mg/kg of diet from 77% to 7% and com-pletely prevented the paralysis that was observed in all animals on the hexachlorophene diet alone. However, in the animals on the combined treatment, histological changes in the brain characteristic of hexachloro-phene were still apparent and the possibility of delayed toxicity beyond the 8 weeks of the experiment could not be eliminated. The protective effect of Aroclor 1254 was explained by its capacity to enhance detoxifica-tion by means of hepatic microsomal enzyme induction (Jones et al., 1974).

7.5 Cytotoxic Effects

Peakall et al. (1972) found a significant increase in chromosome abnormalities in the embryos of ring doves when the parents were fed on a diet containing Aroclor 1254 at 10 mg/kg. Nilsson & Ramel (1974) found no chromosome breakage in *Drosophila melanogaster* when either Clophen A30 or A50 was added to the substrate. Green et al. (1975) administered Aroclor 1242 orally to rats in single doses of 1250, 2500, or 5000 mg/kg or as a repeated dose of 500 mg/kg/day for 4 days. Aroclor 1254 was also administered for 5 days at doses of 75, 150, or 300 mg/kg/day; they found no evidence of a mutagenic potential as assessed by cytogenic analysis of bone marrow and spermatogonia.

7.6 Immunosuppressive Effects

Administration of PCBs leads to an atrophy of lymphoid tissue in chickens (Flick et al., 1965; Vos & Koeman, 1970), in pheasants (Dahlgren et al., 1972), and in rabbits (Vos & Beems, 1971). Vos & de Roij (1972) and Vos & van Driel-Grootenhuis (1972) came to the conclusion that these effects could be attributed to an immunosuppressive effect of PCBs. They found that when guinea pigs fed on diets containing Clophen A60 or Aroclor 1260 at 50 mg/kg were stimulated with tetanus toxoid, a lower antitoxin titre and a lower count of antitoxin-producing cells was obtained than in control guinea pigs, resulting in a significant reduction of immunoglobulins. The skin reaction after tuberculination in animals immunized with Freund's complete adjuvant (as a parameter of cell-mediated immunity) was also depressed at the 50 mg/kg of diet level. Vos & de Roij (1972) suggested that the ability of PCBs to increase the susceptibility of ducklings to duck hepatitis virus (Friend & Trainer, 1970) and of fish to fungal disease (Hansen et al., 1971) could be attributed to this immunosuppressive effect. Kimuru & Baba (1973) found an increased incidence of pneumonia, and lung and intracranial abscesses in rats on a diet containing Kanechlor 400 and suggested that this was due to a lowered resistance to infection.

7.7 Effects on Reproduction

In a one-generation reproduction study, rats were fed with a diet containing Aroclor 1242, 1254, or 1260 at levels of 1, 10, and 100 mg/kg. Decreased survival of pups with Aroclors 1242 and 1254 at 100 mg/kg was noted. No effect on reproduction was detected with Aroclor 1260 (Keplinger et al., 1971). In a two-generation reproduction study (Linder et al., 1974), rats were fed a diet containing Aroclor 1254 at levels of 0, 1, 5, 20, and 100 mg/kg and Aroclor 1260 at levels of 0, 5, 20, and 100 mg/kg. Rats exposed to Aroclor 1254 at dietary levels of 20 mg/kg or more had fewer pups per litter. Aroclor 1260 had no effect on reproduction, even at levels of 100 mg/kg. Kihlström et al. (1973) showed that a daily oral dose of 25 μg of Clophen A60 to female mice for 62 days significantly increased the length of the estrus cycle and decreased the frequency of implanted ova. In order to study the effect of PCBs on the development of sexual functions in the early postnatal period they also mated mice that had been suckled by mothers dosed with Clophen A60 during the lactation period. A decrease in the frequency of implanted ova was noted when both parents of the couple had been suckled with milk containing PCBs.

In the rhesus monkey, Allen (1975) reports a lower fertility and a diminished weight of the young at birth, after the administration of a diet containing Aroclor 1248 at 2.5 mg/kg for several months.

Studies by Aulerich et al. (1971), and Ringer et al. (1972) showed that Aroclor 1254 fed to mink at 5 mg/kg severely affected reproduction.

There have been several reports that PCBs can adversely affect egg production and hatchability in birds. Contamination of feed by PCBs from a heat exchanger was shown to be the cause of reduced hatchability of hen eggs at a large poultry hatchery in the USA (Kolbye, 1972), and this has been confirmed in laboratory experiments. Keplinger et al. (1971) found poor hatchability of eggs from hens receiving diets containing Aroclor 1242 at 10 mg/kg or Aroclor 1254 at 100 mg/kg, but not with hens receiving Aroclor 1260 at 100 mg/kg. An adverse effect on eggs has been noted with Aroclor 1248 at 10 mg/kg (Panel on Hazardous Trace Substances, 1972). Peakall et al. (1972) fed ring doves on a diet containing Aroclor 1254 at 10 mg/kg for 3 months and found a marked reduction in egg hatchability 6 months later, due to embryo mortality.

The viability of salmon eggs bears some relation to their PCB content; Johansson et al. (1970) found a 12% mortality in eggs containing PCBs at the rate of 9.2 mg/kg in extractable fat, and a 100% mortality with 34 mg/kg. Adverse effects on the reproduction of aquatic invertebrates have occurred at water concentrations of PCBs in the region of 5 μg/litre.

The potential teratogenic effect of the PCBs has been studied by dosing pregnant females during the gestation period. No fetal abnormalities were produced in the rat by daily doses of Aroclors 1242, 1254, or 1260 at 10 and 30 mg/kg (Keplinger et al., 1971), or Aroclor 1254 at 100 mg/kg (Villeneuve et al., 1971b), or in the rabbit dosed with Aroclor 1254 at 10 and 50 mg/kg (Villeneuve et al., 1971b). Injection of PCBs into eggs has been reported to produce beak abnormalities in chicks (McLaughlin et al., 1963). Cecil et al. (1974) have claimed that the administration of Aroclors 1232 and 1254 to hens at 20 mg/kg in the diet causes teratogenic effects and a reduction in hatchability of fertile eggs.

7.8 Neoplasia and Adenofibrosis

The liver is the only organ where tumours have been reported following the ingestion of PCBs. Ito et al. (1973) fed groups of 12 male dd mice with diets containing 500, 250, 100 and 0 mg/kg of Kanechlor 500, 400, and 300, respectively. After 1 year, 7/12 mice developed neoplastic nodules (hyperplastic nodules) and 5/12 developed hepatocellular carcinomas, all in mice from the group fed with 500 mg/kg Kanechlor 500. Metastases were not observed. In a second study on mice, combined exposure to Kanechlor 500 and either α- or β-hexachlorocyclohexane isomers enhanced the development of neoplastic nodules (hyperplastic nodules) and hepato-cellular carcinomas. A combination of Kanechlor 500 and γ-hexachlorocyclohexane did not produce tumours. Dosing with Kanechlor 500 alone at a dietary level of 250 mg/kg, and β- or γ-hexachlorocyclohexane at dietary levels of 250, 100 or 50 mg/kg did not produce tumours. However, α-hexachlorocyclohexane produced 8/30 hepatacellular carcinomas and 23/30 hyperplastic nodules.

Groups of 50 BALB/cj male inbred mice were fed dietary concentrations of Aroclor 1254 of 0 or 300 mg/kg (49.8 mg/kg body weight) for 6 or 11 months respectively. No liver tumours were noted in a total of 58 surviving controls. A total of 10 hepatomas (neoplastic or hyperplastic nodules) were noted in 9/22 surviving mice fed Aroclor 1254 for 11 months and in 1/24 surviving mice fed Aroclor 1254 for 6 months. In addition adenofibrosis (cholangiofibrosis) was observed in all 22 livers of mice fed Aroclor 1254 for 11 months, but not in the other groups (Kimbrough & Linder 1974).

In another study (Kimbrough et al., 1975), 200 female Sherman strain COBS random bred rats (descendants of the Osborne Mendel strain) were given a diet containing Aroclor 1260 at 100 mg/kg (11.6–4.3 mg/kg body weight) for approximately 21 months; 200 female rats were kept as controls. The rats were sacrificed when 23 months old. Hepatocellular carcinomas were found in 26/184 of the experimental groups and in 1/173 of the control rats. None of the controls, but 144/184 experimental rats had neoplastic nodules (hyperplastic nodules). Areas of hepatocellular alteration were noted in 28/173 controls and 182/184 experimental rats. No effect of the Aroclor on the incidence of tumours in other organs and no metastases from the liver tumours were observed. In this and two earlier studies, adenofibrosis of the liver was observed in male and female rats fed either Aroclor 1260 or Aroclor 1254 (Kimbrough et al., 1972; 1973); 1975). Adenofibrosis of the liver is a persistent progressive lesion that consists of a marked proliferation of fibrous tissue and epithelial glandular cells which are well differentiated in the mouse but appear atypical in the rat.

In a preliminary study, liver tumours (multiple adenomatous nodules) were induced by Kanechlor 400 in 6/10 female, but not in male Donryu rats. The dietary exposure varied throughout the study and the number of animals used was small (10 experimental and 5 control rats for each sex) (Kimura & Baba, 1973). Makiura et al. (1974) reported that PCBs (Kanechlor 500) inhibited the induction of liver tumours in male Sprague-Dawley rats by the known carcinogens 3′ methyl-p-dimethylaminoazobenzene, N-2-fluosenyl acetamide, and diethylnitrosamine.

8. EFFECTS OF PCBs AND PCTs ON MAN—
EPIDEMIOLOGICAL AND CLINICAL STUDIES

In June 1968, patients appeared at the Dermatology Clinic of Kyushu University Hospital, Fukuoka, Japan suffering from chloracne. A group at the University undertook intensive clinical, chemical, and epidemiological investigations and found that the disease originated from the consumption of a batch of rice oil supplied in February 1968; the disease was called Yusho (rice oil disease) (Katsuki, 1969). This batch of rice oil was found to be contaminated with Kanechlor 400, a 48% chlorinated biphenyl, at 2000–3000 mg/kg which entered the oil through a leak in a heat exchanger (Tsukamoto et al., 1969). The symptoms and signs of Yusho were described by Goto & Higuchi (1969) and by Okumura & Katsuki (1969). The earliest signs were enlargement and hypersecretion of the Meibomian glands of the eyes, swelling of the eylids, and pigmentation of the nails and mucous membranes, occasionally associated with fatigue, nausea, and vomiting. This was usually followed by hyperkeratosis and darkening of the skin with follicular enlargement and acneform eruptions, frequently with a secondary staphylococcal infection. These skin changes were most often seen on the neck and upper chest, but in severe cases extended to the whole body. Biopsy skin samples showed hyperkeratosis, dilation of the follicles, and an accumulation of melanin in the basal cells of the epidermis; melanin granules have also been observed in biopsy samples of the conjunctiva. Oedema of the arms and legs was seen in some patients. There were no definite signs of liver enlargement or liver disorders (Okumura & Katsuki 1969), but slight rises in serum transaminases and in alkaline phosphatase were detected, and a liver sample from a Yusho patient showed an increase in the smooth endoplasmic reticulum (Hirayama et al., 1969). The majority of the patients were found to have respiratory symptoms, and suffered from a chronic bronchitis-like disturbance that persisted for several years (Shigematsu et al., 1971, 1974).

Yusho patients did not appear to suffer from central nervous effects, but some complained of numbness of the arms and legs. Murai & Kuroiwa (1971) found a decrease in the conduction velocity in peripheral sensory nerves.

Yoshimura (1971) reported diminished growth in boys but not in girls, who consumed the oil. Babies born to Yusho mothers were smaller than normal. Newborn babies showed a dark brown skin pigmentation, which disappeared after a few months (Yagamuchi et al., 1971; Taki et al., 1969). Funatsu et al. (1972) found spotted and sporadic ossification of the skull and facial oedema with exophthalmia in four babies, but there was no evidence of any teratogenic action.

Determinations of PCB concentrations in the tissue of Yusho patients were made several months after the ingestion of the oil, apparently by an X-ray fluorescence method for organic chlorine (Goto & Higuchi, 1969). Abdominal fat contained 13.1 mg/kg, subcutaneous fat 75.5 mg/kg, and nails 59 mg/kg. The mesenteric adipose tissue in six Yusho patients, analysed by gas–liquid chromatography 1–3 years after the occurrence of intoxication, contained PCB levels of 2.5 mg/kg on average, which was considerably higher than the normal value. (Masuda et al., 1974a). The mean blood level of PCBs in patients was 0.6 or 0.7 µg/100 ml (0.3 µg/100 ml for the general population) five years after exposure (Masuda et al., 1974b; Takamatsu et al., 1974). These authors also noted a specific gas–liquid chromatographic pattern, peculiar to Yusho patients, which is still observed.

Hirayama et al. (1974) also reported that the serum bilirubin level of patients was significantly lower than the normal level and was negatively correlated with the blood level of PCBs and the serum triglyceride level.

A considerable number of patients had elevated serum triglyceride levels, up to four times the normal values, although this was not correlated with the severity of the symptoms; these high values were maintained for three years in many patients (Uzawa, 1972). There were no marked abnormalities in serum cholesterol and phospholipid levels (Okumura & Katsuki, 1969; Uzawa et al., 1969). Nagai et al. (1969) reported an increase in urinary 17-ketosteroid excretion. Kusuda (1971) also observed changes in the menstrual cycle in approximately 60% of 81 female Yusho patients as compared with their cycles prior to exposure. Okumura et al. (1974) examined the relationship between the blood levels of triglycerides and PCBs in 42 patients and observed a positive correlation. Uzawa et al. (1972) showed that high values of serum triglycerides were maintained for 3 years in many patients. Shigematsu et al. (1971) examined serum immunoglobulin levels in 38 patients, 2 years after onset, and observed a decrease in IgA and IgM and an increase in IgG. Saito et al. (1972) reported lower IgM levels in patients showing chloracne.

Urabe (1974) reported that the total number of Yusho patients had reached 1200 by 13 September 1973 and that 22 of them had died. Muco-cutaneous signs had decreased year by year, but neurological and respiratory signs and symptoms and various complaints such as general fatigue, anorexia, abdominal pain, and headache had become more prominent among the patients. The smallest amount of oil that produced symptoms when ingested over approximately 120 days, contained approximately 0.5 g of PCBs, or approximately 0.07 mg/kg body weight per day (Kuratsune, 1972a). Recently chlorinated dibenzofurans at 5 mg/kg were found in three samples of the toxic rice oil that contained PCB levels of about 1000 mg/kg (Nagayama et al., 1975).

Symptoms similar to those of Yusho have been observed in workers in a Japanese condenser factory, including pigmentation of the fingers and, nails, and acneiform eruptions on the jaw, back, and thighs. It was thought that these effects arose from local contact with PCBs; when the use of PCBs ceased, the symptoms disappeared (Hasegawa et al., 1972b).

9. EVALUATION OF HEALTH RISKS TO MAN FROM EXPOSURE TO PCBs AND PCTs

9.1 Species Variation

The data in sections 7 and 8 indicate that man appears to be the species most sensitive to PCBs, the consumption of relatively small amounts having resulted in a severe disease (Yusho) in 1200 persons in Japan. The monkey is the only experimental species in which effects qualitatively and quantitatively approaching those in man have been observed; Allen (1975) attributed this to metabolic differences leading to a slower elimination than that observed in other species tested.

Conclusions concerning the specific effects of PCBs on different species are confused by uncertainty arising from the presence of toxic impurities.

The rice oil that caused the outbreak of Yusho was contaminated with PCBs containing relatively high amounts of tetrachlorodibenzofuran (see section 8), but the sample used in the monkey experiments had a low content of these impurities, so it is not clear whether PCBs alone were responsible for the Yusho incident. Further uncertainty arises from reports from Finland of high PCB concentrations in blood and body fat of occupationally exposed workers with no indication of adverse effects, while at similar tissue concentrations Japanese workers showed skin lesions typical of Yusho (see section 5.5.3).

A species-specific toxic manifestation that can probably be attributed to toxic impurities, is the abdominal oedema and hydropericardium seen in birds affected by some commercial PCB mixtures.

Mink is another species showing a high sensitivity to PCBs. Deaths have been produced with diets containing PCB levels of 30 mg/kg; no information is available on any species-specific metabolic pathway in the mink that would account for this susceptibility.

9.2 Dose–Effect Relationships

The following is a summary of the data in Sections 7 and 8 concerning the relationship between mammalian toxicity and dose. Approximate calculations of the daily dose in mg/kg body weight derived from the dietary concentration are given in parentheses.[a]

9.2.1 Body weight

Body weight was reduced in rats after 8 months of dietary intake of Aroclor 1254 at 100 mg/kg (corresponding to 5 mg/kg body weight); no effects were observed at 20 mg/kg in the diet (corresponding to 1 mg/kg body weight).

Dose-dependent retardation of weight gain was observed in mink after 4 months of dietary intake of Aroclor 1254 at 5 and 10 mg/kg (corresponding to 0.5 and 1.1 mg/kg body weight respectively).

9.2.2 Effects on liver

Liver weight

Dose-dependent increase in liver weight was observed in rats receiving Aroclors 1242, 1254 and 1260 at concentrations of more than 20 mg/kg

---

[a] When no food consumption figures were available from the experimental studies, the following factors were used to transform mg/kg in the diet to mg/kg body weight: mouse (7), rat (20), guinea-pig (25), mink (10), rabbit (33), monkey (25).

in the diet (corresponding to >1.4 mg/kg body weight). Male rats were more sensitive than female rats; no effects were observed with Aroclors 1254 and 1260 at concentrations lower than 20 mg/kg in the diet (corresponding to <1.4 mg/kg body weight). Effects were less marked with the lower chlorinated PCBs.

Liver changes

Smooth endoplasmic reticulum proliferation with fat droplet inclusions were observed in the liver tissue of rats after 8 months of dietary intake of Aroclor 1254 at 20 mg/kg (corresponding to 1.4 mg/kg body weight).

Liver damage was observed with Aroclors 1242 and 1254 in rabbits receiving 14 weekly oral doses of 150 mg/kg body weight; no effect was observed with Aroclor 1221.

Liver enzyme activity[a]

Increase in microsomal enzyme activity was observed in male rats after 8 months of dietary intake of Aroclor 1254 of 20 mg/kg (corresponding to 1 mg/kg body weight). No effect was observed at 2 mg/kg in the diet (corresponding to 0.1 mg/kg body weight). Effects were less marked in female rats.

Increased activity was also observed with Aroclors 1242 and 1016 in male rats receiving 21 daily oral doses of 1 mg/kg body weight.

Liver porphyria

Effects were observed in rats after several months of dietary intake of Aroclor 1254 at 100 mg/kg (corresponding to 5 mg/kg body weight); dose-dependent effects were observed in female rats after 21 daily oral doses of Aroclor 1242 at 10 and 100 mg/kg; no effects were noted at 1 mg/kg body weight.

Liver vitamin A

Reduction of hepatic vitamin A was observed in rats receiving Aroclor 1242 at the rate of 100 mg/kg in the diet (corresponding to 5 mg/kg body weight).

Liver tumours

Hepatocellular carcinomas were observed in mice after one year of dietary intake of Kaneclor 500 at 500 mg/kg (corresponding to 75 mg/kg

---

[a] According to Litterst, et al. (1972) the dose producing an effect on nitroreductase activity in the rat corresponds to 0.5 mg/kg in the diet (corresponding to 0.3 mg/kg body weight).

body weight); no carcinomas were observed with Kaneclor 500 at 250 mg/kg in the diet (corresponding to 37.5 mg/kg body weight), or with Kaneclor 300 and 400 at 500 mg/kg in the diet (corresponding to 75 mg/kg body weight).

Hepatomas were observed in mice after 10 months of daily intake of Aroclor 1254 at 300 mg/kg in the diet (corresponding to 49.8 mg/kg body weight).

Hepatocellular carcinomas were observed in rats after 21 months of daily intake of Aroclor 1260 at 100 mg/kg in the diet (corresponding to 11.6–4.3 mg/kg body weight).

9.2.3   Reproduction

Effects on reproduction were observed in the mouse at a daily oral dose of 0.025 mg Clophen A60; in the rat at a dietary level of Aroclor 1254 of 20 mg/kg (corresponding to 1 mg/kg body weight) with the effects decreasing with higher chlorinated PCBs; in the mink at a dietary level of Aroclor 1254 of 5 mg/kg (corresponding to 0.5 mg/kg body weight); and in the monkey at a dietary level of Aroclor 1248 of 2.5 mg/kg (corresponding to 0.1 mg/kg body weight).

9.2.4   Immunosuppression

Immunosuppressive effects were observed in the guinea-pig at a dietary level of Clophen A60 or Aroclor 1260 of 50 mg/kg (corresponding to 2 mg/kg body weight).

9.2.5   Skin effects

In man, symptoms of Yusho disease were observed at a dietary level of 4.2 mg/day of PCBs (corresponding to 0.07 mg/kg body weight/day for a 60-kg person). A value of 0.50 g was estimated as the quantity of PCBs consumed over approximately 120 days above which toxic symptoms were evident. Similar effects were observed in the monkey at a dietary level of Aroclor 1248 of 2.5 mg/kg (corresponding to 0.1 mg/kg body weight) after several months.

9.3   Nondetected effect levels

The assessment of non detected effect levels for toxic effects is complicated by the different activities of the component PCBs and by the presence of impurities, in addition to the influence of inter- and intraspecies variation, age, sex, and length of exposure. Moreover, many of the available experimental studies do not include a nondetected effect level.

The most sensitive species appears to be man, and effects have been observed at intake rates of 0.07 mg/kg body weight/day. This may have been influenced by the intake of impurities more toxic than PCBs, but similar effects have been produced in the monkey, at the same order of dosage, with a product containing little of these impurities. At this dosage level, no effects may be expected on growth, liver enlargement, and liver enzyme activity in less sensitive species such as the rat. Although non-detected effect levels are not available for effects on immunosuppression and reproduction, and for certain biochemical effects on the liver, it seems unlikely that these effects would be apparent at intake rates of 0.1 mg/kg body weight/day. Carcinogenic effects have been observed in rats and mice at doses two orders of magnitude greater than this, but there is no epidemiological evidence to suggest that PCBs cause tumours in man. According to Grant et al. (1974) rats fed on a diet containing Aroclor at the rate of 2 mg/kg (equivalent to about 0.1 mg/kg body weight) showed PCB levels of 8 μg/100 ml in blood and 26.1 mg/kg in body fat. However, values much higher than these have been observed in men occupationally exposed to PCBs without evidence of any toxic effects (see section 5.5.3).

It is not possible at present to resolve this conflict in the evidence on the toxicity of PCBs to man.

ABBOT, D. C., COLLINS, G. B. & GOULDING, R. (1972) Organochlorine pesticide residues in human fat in the United Kingdom 1969–71. *Br. med. J.*, **2**: 553–556.

ACKER, L. & SCHULTE, E. (1970) Über das Vorkommen von chlorierten Biphenylen und Hexachlorbenzol neben chlorierten Insektiziden in Humanmilch und menschlichem Fettgewebe. *Naturwissenschaften*, **57**: 497 (in German).

ACKER, L. & SCHULTE, E. (1974) Chlorkohlenwasserstoffe in menschlichem Fettgewebe, *Naturwissenschaften*, **61**: 1–4 (in German).

ADDISON, R. F., FLETCHER, G. L., RAY, S. & DOANE, J. (1972) Analysis of a chlorinated terphenyl (Aroclor 5460) and its deposition in tissues of the cod (*Gadus morhua*). *Bull. environ. Contam. Toxicol.*, **8**: 52–60.

AHLING, B. & JENSEN, S. (1970) Reversed liquid–liquid partition in determination of polychlorinated biphenyl (PCB) and chlorinated pesticides in water. *Anal. Chem.*, **42**: 1483–1486.

AHMED, M. & FOCHT, D. D. (1973) Degradation of polychlorinated biphenyls by two species of *Achromobacter*. *Can. J. Microbiol.*, **19**: 47–52.

AHNOFF, M. & JOSEFSSON, B. (1973) Confirmation studies on polychlorinated biphenyls (PCB) from river waters using mass fragmentography. *Anal. Lett.*, **6**: 1083–1093.

AHNOFF, M. & JOSEFSSON, B. (1974) Simple apparatus for on-site continuous liquid–liquid extraction of organic compounds from natural waters. *Anal. Chem.*, **46**: 658–663.

AHNOFF, M. & JOSEFSSON, B. (1975) Clean-up procedures for PCB analysis on river water extracts. *Bull. environ. Contam. Toxicol.*, **13**: 159–166.

ALBRO, P. W. & FISHBEIN, L. (1972) Intestinal absorption of polychlorinated biphenyls in rats. *Bull. environ. Contam. Toxicol.*, **8**: 26–31.

ALLEN, J. R. (1975) Response of the non-human primate to polychlorinated biphenyl exposure. *Fed. Proc.*, **34**: 1675–1679.

ALLEN, J. R., ABRAHAMSON, L. J. & NORBACK, D. H. (1973) Biological effects of polychlorinated biphenyls and triphenyls on the subhuman primate. *Environ. Res.*, **6**: 344–354.

ALLEN, J. R. & NORBACK, D. A. (1973) Polychlorinated biphenyl- and triphenyl-induced mucosal hyperplasia in primates. *Science*, **179**: 498–499.

ALLEN, J. R., CARSTENS, L. A. & BARSOTTI, D. A. (1974) Residual effects of short-term, low-level exposure of non-human primates to polychlorinated biphenyls. *Toxicol. appl. Pharmacol.*, **30**: 440–451.

ALVARES, A. P. & KAPPAS, A. (1975) Induction of aryl hydrocarbon hydroxylase by chlorinated biphenyls in the foeto-placental unit and in neonatal livers during lactation. *FEBS Lett.*, **50**: 172–174.

ARMOUR, J. A. & BURKE, J. A. (1970) Method for separating polychlorinated biphenyls from DDT and its analogs. *J. Assoc. Off. Anal. Chem.*, **53**: 761–768.

AULERICH, R. J., RINGER, R. K., SEAGRAN, H. L. & YOUATT, W. G. (1971) Effects of feeding coho salmon and other Great Lakes fish on mink reproduction. *Can. J. Zool.*, **49**: 611–616.

AULERICH, R. J., RINGER, R. K. & IWAMOTO, S. (1973) Reproductive failure and mortality in mink fed on Great Lake fish. *J. Reprod. Fertil.*, **19** (Suppl.): 365–376.

BAGLEY, G. E., REICHEL, W. L. & CROMARTIE, E. (1970) Identification of polychlorinated biphenyls in two bald eagles by combined gas–liquid chromatography–mass spectroscopy. *J. Assoc. Off. Anal. Chem.*, **53**: 251–261.

BAILEY, S. & BUNYAN, P. J. (1972) Interpretation of persistence and effects of polychlorinated biphenyls in birds. *Nature (Lond.)*, **236**: 34–36.

BASTOMSKY, C. H., SOLYMOSS, B., ZSIGMOND, G. & WYSE, J. M. (1975) On the mechanism of polychlorinated biphenyl-induced hypobilirubinaemia. *Clin. chim. Acta*, **61**: 171–174.

BAUER, H., SCHULZ, K. H. & SPIEGELBERG, U. (1961) Berufliche Vergiftungen bei der

Herstellung von Chlorphenol-Verbindungen. *Arch. Gewerbepathol. Gewerbehyg.*, **18**: 538–555.

BENTHE, H. F., KNOP, J. & SCHMOLDT, A. (1972a) Absorption and distribution of polychlorinated biphenyls (PCB) after inhalatory application. *Arch. Toxikol.*, **29**: 85–95 (in German).

BENTHE, H. F., SCHMOLDT, A. & SCHMIDT, H. (1972b) Induction of microsomal liver enzymes after polychlorinated biphenyls (PCB) and following stress. *Arch. Toxikol.*, **29**; 97–106 (in German).

BERG, O. W., DIOSADY, P. L. & REES, G. A. V. (1972) Column chromatographic separation of polychlorinated biphenyls from chlorinated hydrocarbon pesticides and their subsequent gas chromatographic quantitation in terms of derivatives. *Bull. environ. Contam. Toxicol.*, **7**: 338–347.

BERGLUND, F. (1972) Levels of polychlorinated biphenyls in foods in Sweden. *Environ. Health Perspect*, **1**: 67–69.

BERLIN, M., GAGE, J. C. & HOLM, S. (1973) *The metabolism and distribution of 2,4,5,2′,5′-pentachlorobiphenyl in the mouse.* In : *PCB Conference II.* National Swedish Environment Protection Board Publications: 4E, pp. 101–107.

BERLIN, M., GAGE, J. C. & HOLM, S. (1974) *Distribution and metabolism of polychlorobiphenyls.* In : *Proceedings of the International Symposium on Recent Advances in Environmental Pollution, Paris, 24–28 June.* pp. 8.

BERLIN, M., GAGE, J. & HOLM, S. (1975) The distribution and metabolism of 2,4,5,2′,5′-pentachlorobiphenyl. *Arch. environ. Health*, **30**: 141–147.

BICKERS, D. R., HARBER, L. C., KAPPAS, A. & ALVARES, A. P. (1972) Polychlorinated biphenyls: comparative effects of high and low chlorine containing Aroclors on hepatic mixed function oxidase. *Res, Comm. Chem. Pathol. Pharmacol.*, **3**: 505–511.

BIDLEMAN, T. F. & OLNEY, C. E. (1974) High-volume collection of atmospheric polychlorinated biphenyls. *Bull. environ. Contam. Toxicol.*, **11**: 442–450.

BITMAN, J., CECIL, H. C. & HARRIS, S. J. (1972) Biological effects of polychlorinated biphenyl in rats and quail. *Environ. Health Perspec.*, **1**: 145–149.

BJERK, J. E. (1972) Rester av DDT og polyklorerte bifenyler i Norsk humant materiale. *Tidsskr. Nor-Laegeforen.*, **92**: 15–19 (cited by Kimbrough, 1974).

BOURNE, W. P. P. & BOGEN, A. A. (1972) Polychlorinated biphenyls in North Atlantic seabirds, *Mar. Pollut. Bull.*, **3** (11): 172–175.

BOWES, G. W., MULVIHILL, M. J., SIMONEIT, B. R. T., BURLINGAME, A. L. & RISEBROUGH, R. W. (1975) Identification of chlorinated dibenzofurans in American polychlorinated biphenyls. *Nature (Lond.)*, **256**, 305–307.

BROADHURST, M. G. (1972) Use and replaceability of polychlorinated biphenyls. *Environ. Health Perspect.*, **2**: 81–102.

BRUCKNER, J. V., KHANNA, K. L. & CORNISH, H. H. (1973) Biological responses of the rat to polychlorinated biphenyls. *Toxicol. appl. Pharmacol.*, **24**: 434–448.

BRUGGEMAN, VON J., BUSCH, L., DRESCHER-KADAN, U., EISELI, W. & HOPPE, P. (1974) Pesticid—und PCB—Ruckstunde in Organen von Wildtieren als Indikatoren für Umweltkontamination. *Z. Jagdwiss.*, **20**: 70–74.

BURSE, V. W., KIMBROUGH, R. D., VILLANUEVAS, E. C., JENNINGS, R. W., LINDER, R. E. & SOVOCOOL, G. W. (1974) Polychlorinated biphenyls. Storage, distribution, excretion and recovery: liver morphology after prolonged dietary ingestion. *Arch. environ. Health*, **29**: 301–307.

CARNES, R. A., DOERGER, J. U. & SPARKS, H. L. (1973) Polychlorinated biphenyls in solid waste and solid-waste-related materials. *Arch. environ. Contam. Toxicol.*, **1**: 27–35.

CECIL, H. C., HARRIS, S. J., BITMAN, J. & FRIES, G. F. (1973) Polychlorinated biphenyl-induced decrease in liver vitamin A in Japanese quail and rats. *Bull. environ. Contam. Toxicol.*, **9**: 179–185.

CECIL, H. C., BITMAN, J., LILLIE, R. J., FRIES, G. F. & VERRETT, J. (1974) Embryotoxic and teratogenic effects in unhatched fertile eggs from hens fed polychlorinated biphenyls (PCBs). *Bull. environ. Contam. Toxicol.*, **11**: 489–495.

CECIL, H. C., HARRIS, S. J. & BITMAN, J. (1975) Effects of polychlorinated biphenyls and terphenyls and polybrominated biphenyls on pentobarbital sleeping times of Japanese quail. *Arch. environ. Contam. Toxicol.,* **3**, 183–192.

CHOI, P. S. K., NACK, H. & FLINN, J. E. (1974) Distribution of polychlorinated biphenyls in an aerated biological oxidation wastewater treatment system. *Bull. environ. Contam. Toxicol.,* **11**: 12–17.

CLAUS, B. & ACKER, L. (1975) Zur Kontamination von Milch und Milcherzeugnissen mit chlorierten Kohlenwasserstoffen im Westphälischen Raum II Ergebnisse und Diskussion. *Zeitschrift fur Lebensmitteluntersuchung und forschung,* **159** (3): 129–137.

COLLINS, G. B., HOLMES, D. C. & JACKSON, F. J. (1972) The estimation of polychlorobiphenyls. *J. Chromatogr.,* **71**: 443–449.

COMMISSION OF THE EUROPEAN COMMUNITIES (1974) *European Colloquium. Problems raised by the contamination of man and his environment by persistent pesticides and organohalogenated compounds.* Luxembourg, 14–16 May 1964.

COOLEY, N. R., KELTNER, J. M. & FORESTER, J. (1972) Mirex and Aroclor 1254: effect on accumulation by *Tetrahymena pyriformis* strain W. *J. Protozool.,* **19**: 636–638.

CURLEY, A., BURSE, V. W., GRIM, M. E., JENNINGS, R. W. & LINDER, R. E. (1971) Polychlorinated biphenyls: distribution and storage in body fluids and tissues of Sherman rats. *Environ. Res.,* **4**: 481–495.

CURLEY, A., BURSE, V. W. & GRIM, M. E. (1973a) Polychlorinated biphenyls: evidence of transplacental passage in the Sherman rat. *Fd. cosmet. Toxicol.,* **11**: 471–476.

CURLEY, A., BURSE, V. W., JENNINGS, R. W., VILLANUEVA, E. C., TOMATIS, L. & AKAZAKI, K. (1973b) Chlorinated hydrocarbon pesticides and related compounds in adipose tissue from people of Japan. *Nature (Lond),* **242**: 338–340.

CURLEY, A., BURSE, W. V., JENNINGS, R. W., VILLANUEVA, E. C. & KIMBROUGH, R. D. (1975) Evidence of tetrachlorodibenzofuran (TCDF) in Aroclor 1254 and the urine of rats following dietary exposure to Aroclor 1254. *Bull. environ. Contam. Toxicol.,* **14**: 153–158.

DAHLGREN, R. B., GREICHUS, Y. A. & LINDER, R. L. (1971) Storage and excretion of polychlorinated biphenyls in the pheasant. *J. Wildlife Manag.,* **35**: 823–828.

DAHLGREN, R. B., LINDER, R. L. & CARLSON, C. W. (1972) Polychlorinated biphenyls: their effects on penned pheasants. *Environ. Health Perspect.,* **1**: 89–101.

DE FREITAS, A. S. & NORSTROM, R. J. (1974) Turnover and metabolism of polychlorinated biphenyls in relation to their chemical structure and the movement of lipids in the pigeon. *Can. J. Physiol. Pharmacol.,* **52**: 1080–1094.

DEPARTMENT OF HEALTH EDUCATION AND WELFARE (1972) *Environ. Health Perspect.* Experimental Issue 1, April 1972. DHEW, Bethesda, MD, USA. *Publ. No. (NIH) 72–218.*

DE VOS, R. H. & PEET, E. W. (1971) Thin-layer chromatography of polychlorinated biphenyls. *Bull. environ. Contam. Toxicol.,* **6**: 164–170.

DOGUCHI, M. & FUKANO, S. (1975) Residue levels of polychlorinated terphenyls, polychlorinated biphenyls and DDT in human blood. *Bull. environ. Contam. Toxicol.,* **13**: 57–63.

DOGUCHI, M., FUKANO, S. & USHIO, F. (1974) Polychlorinated terphenyls in the human fat. *Bull. environ. Contam. Toxicol.,* **11** (2): 157–158.

DUKE, T. W., LOWE, J. I. & WILSON, A. J. JR (1970) A polychlorinated biphenyl (Aroclor 1254) in the water, sediment and biota of Escambia Bay, Florida. *Bull. environ. Contam. Toxicol.,* **5**: 171–180.

ECOBICHON, D. J. & COMEAU, A. M. (1974) Comparative effects of commercial Aroclors on rat liver enzyme activities. *Chem.-Biol. Interactions,* **9**: 341–350.

EKSTEDT, J. & ODEN, S. (1974) *Chlorinated hydrocarbons in the lower atmosphere in Sweden.* Report from Department of Soil Science, Royal Agricultural College, S–75007, Uppsala 7. pp. 1–16.

ENVIRONMENTAL SANITATION BUREAU, MINISTRY OF HEALTH & WELFARE (1973) *Survey on foods contamination.* Report of comprehensive investigation on the prevention of pollution by PCBs, 191–210 (in Japanese).

FINKLEA, J., PRIESTER, L. E., CREASON, J. P., HAUSER, T., HINNERS, T. & HAMMER, D. I.

(1972) Polychlorinated biphenyl residues in human plasma expose a major urban pollution problem. *Am. J. pub. Health*, **62**: 645–651.

FISHER, N. S., GRAHAM, L. B., CARPENTER, E. J. & WURSTER, C. F. (1972) Geographic differences in phytoplankton sensitivity to PCBs. *Nature (Lond.)*, **241**: 548–549.

FLICK, D. F., O'DELL, R. G. & CHILDS, V. A. (1965) Studies of the chick edema disease. 3. Similarity of symptoms produced by feeding chlorinated biphenyl. *Poult. Sci.*, **44**: 1460–1465.

FREUDENTHAL, J. & GREVE, P. A. (1973) Polychlorinated terphenyls in the environment. *Bull. environ. Contam. Toxicol.*, **10**: 108–111.

FRIEND, M. & TRAINER, D. O. (1970) Polychlorinated biphenyl: interaction with duck hepatitis virus. *Science*, **170**: 1314–1316.

FRIES, G. F., MARROW, G. S. JR & GORDON, C. H. (1973) Long-term studies of residue retention and excretion by cows fed a polychlorinated biphenyl (Aroclor 1254). *J. agr. Food Chem.*, **21**: 117–121.

FUJITA, S., TZUJI, H., KATO, K., SAEKI, S. & TSUKAMOTO, H. (1971) Effect of biphenyl chlorides on rat liver microsomes. *Fukuoka med. Acta.*, **62**: 30–34.

FUKADA, K., INUYAMA, Y., TAKESHITA, T. & YAMAMOTO, S. (1973) Present state of environmental pollution by PCB in Shimane Prefecture. *Shimare Igaku*, **5**: 1–25 (in Japanese).

FUKANO, S., USHIO, F. & DOGUCHI, M. (1974) PCB, PCT and pesticides residues in fish collected from the Tama River. *Ann. Rep. Tokyo Metr. Res. Lab. P.H.*, **25**: 297–305 (in Japanese).

FUNATSU, I., YAMASHITA, F., ITO, Y., TZUGAWA, S., FUNATSU, T., YOSHIKANE, T., HAYASHI, M., KATO, T., YAKUSHIJI, M., OKAMOTO, G., YAMASAKI, S., ARIMA, T., KUNO, T., IDE, H. & IBE, I. (1972) PCB induced fetopathy. I. Clinical observation. *Kurume med. J.*, **19**: 43–51 (in English).

GARDNER, A. M., CHEN, J. F., ROACH, J. A. G. & RAEGLIS, E. P. (1973) Polychlorinated biphenyls. Hydroxylated urinary metabolites of 2,5,2′,5′-tetrachlorobiphenyl identified in rabbits. *Biochem. biophys. res. Commun.*, **55**: 1377–1384.

GILBERTSON, M. & REYNOLDS, L. (1974) *DDE and PCB in Canadian wild birds*. In: *Occasional paper, Canadian Wildlife Service, Environment*, Canada, Ottawa, pp. 1–16.

GOLDSTEIN, J. A., HICKMAN, P. & JUE, D. L. (1974) Experimental hepatic porphyria induced by polychlorinated biphenyls. *Toxicol. appl. Pharmacol.*, **27**: 437–448.

GOLDSTEIN, J. A., MCKINNEY, J. D., LUCIEN, G. W., MOORE, J. A., HICKMAN, P. & BERGMAN, H. (1975a) Effects of hexachlorobiphenyl isomers and 2,3,7,8-tetrachlorodibenzofuran (TCDF) on hepatic drug metabolism and porphyria accumulation. *Pharmacologist*, **16**: 239 (Abstract No. 278).

GOLDSTEIN, J. A., HICKMAN, P., BURSE, V. W. & BERGMAN, H. (1975b) A comparative study of two polychlorinated biphenyl mixture (Aroclor 1242 and 1016) containing 42% chlorine on induction of hepatic porphyria and drug metabolizing enzymes. *Toxicol. appl. Pharmacol.*, **32**: 461–473.

GOTO, M. & HIGUCHI, K. (1969) The symptomatology of Yusho (chlorobiphenyls poisoning) in dermatology. *Fuoka Act. Med.*, **60**: 409–431.

GRANT, D. L., MOODIE, C. A. & PHILLIPS, W. E. J. (1974) Toxicodynamics of Aroclor 1254 in the male rat. *Environ. physiol. Biochem.*, **4**: 214–225.

GRANT, D. L. & PHILLIPS, W. E. J. (1974) The effect of age and sex on the toxicity of Aroclor 1254, a polychlorinated biphenyl, in the rat. *Bull. environ. Contam. Toxicol.*, **12**: 145–152.

GRANT, D. L., PHILLIPS, W. E. J. & VILLENEUVE, D. C. (1971a) Metabolism of a polychlorinated biphenyl (Aroclor 1254) mixture in the rat. *Bull. environ. Contam. Toxicol.*, **6**: 102–112.

GRANT, D. L., VILLENEUVE, D. C., MCCULLY, K. A. & PHILLIPS, W. E. J. (1971b) Placental transfer of polychlorinated biphenyls in the rabbit. *Environ. Physiol.*, **1**: 61–66.

GREEN, S. G., CARR, J. V., PALMER, K. A. & OSWALD, E. J. (1975) Lack of cytogenetic effects in bone marrow and spermatagonial cells in rats treated with polychlorinated biphenyls (Aroclor 1242 and 1254). *Bull. environ. Contam. Toxicol.*, **13**: 14–22.

HAMMER, D. I., FINKLEA, J. F., PRIESTER, L. E., KEIL, J. E., SANDIFER, S. H. & BRIDBORN, K.

(1972) Polychlorinated biphenyl residues in the plasma and hair of refuse workers. *Environ. Health Perspect.,* **1** (15): 83.

HAMMOND, A. L. (1972) Chemical pollution: polychlorinated biphenyls. *Science,* **175**: 155–156.

HANSEN, D. J., PARRISH, P. R., LOWE, J. I., WILSON, A. J. JR & WILSON, P. D. (1971) Chronic toxicity, uptake and retention of Aroclor 1254 in two estuarine fishes. *Bull. environ. Contam. Toxicol.,* **6**: 113–119.

HAQUE, R., SCHMEDDING, D. W. & FREED, V. H. (1974) Aqueous solubility, absorption and vapour behaviour of polychlorinated biphenyl Aroclor 1254. *Environ. Sci. Technol.,* **8**: 139–142.

HARA, I., HARADA, H., KIMURA, S., ENDO, T. & KAWANO, K. (1974) Follow up health examination in an electric condenser factory after cessation of PCBs usage (1st report) *Jpn. J. Ind. Health,* **16**: 365–366 (in Japanese).

HARVEY, G. R. & STEINHAUER, W. G. (1974) Atmospheric transport of polychlorobiphenyls to the North Atlantic. *Atmos. Environ.,* **8**: 777–782.

HARVEY, G. R., STEINHAUER, W. G. & TEAL, J. M. (1973) Polychlorobiphenyls in North Atlantic Ocean water. *Science,* **180**: 643–644.

HASEGAWA, H., SATO, M. & TSURUTA, H. (1972a) PCBs concentration in the blood of workers handling PCB. *Occup. Health,* **10**: 50–55 (in Japanese).

HASEGAWA, H., SATO, M. & TSURUTA, H. (1972b) *PCB concentration in air of PCB-using plants and health examination of workers* (in Japanese). In: *Report on Special Research on Prevention of Environmental Pollution by PCB-like Substances.* Tokyo, Research Co-ordination Bureau, Science and Technology Agency, pp. 141–149.

HEATH, R. G., SPANN, J. W., KREITZER, J. F. & VANCE, C. (1970) *Effects of polychlorinated biphenyls on birds* In: *Proceedings of the 15th Congress of International. Ornithology, The Hague,* pp. 475–485.

HESSELBERG, R. J. & SCHERR, D. D. (1974) PCBs and *p,p′* DDE in the blood of cachectic patients. *Bull. environ. Contam. Toxicol.,* **11**: 202–205.

HIRAYAMA, C., IRISA, T. & YAMAMOTO, T. (1969) Fine structural changes of the liver in a patient with chlorobiphenyls intoxication. *Fukuoka Acta Med.,* **60**: 455–461 (in Japanese).

HIRAYAMA, C., OKUMURA, M., NAGAI, J. & MASUDA, Y. (1974) Hypobilirubinemia in patients with polychlorinated biphenyls poisoning. *Clin. chim. Acta.,* **55**: 97–100.

HOLDGATE, M. W. (1971) *The sea bird wreck in the Irish Sea, Autumn 1969.* Natural Environmental Research Council (Publication Series C4).

HOLDEN, A. V. (1970a) International co-operative study of organochlorine pesticide residues in terrestial and aquatic wildlife 1967/1968. *Pest. monit. J.,* **4**: 117–135.

HOLDEN, A. V. (1970b) Source of polychlorinated biphenyl contamination in the marine environment. *Nature (Lond.),* **228**: 1220–1221.

HOLDEN, A. V. (1973a) International co-operative study of organochlorine and mercury residues in wildlife, 1969–71. *Pest. monit. J.,* **7**: 37–52.

HOLDEN, A. V. (1973b) *Monitoring PCBs in water and wildlife.* In: *PCB Conference II,* Stockholm, *Swedish Environment Protection Board,* Publication: **4E**, pp. 23–33.

HOLDEN, A. V. & MARSDEN, K. (1969) Single-stage clean-up of animal tissue extracts for organochlorine residue analysis. *J. Chromatogr.,* **44**: 481–492.

HUTZINGER, O., JAMIESON, W. D., SAFE, S., PAULMANN, L. & AM⌐ , R. (1974) Identification of metabolic dechlorination of highly chlorinated bipheny ⌐bit. *Nature (Lond.),* **252**: 698–699.

HUTZINGER, O., NASH, D. M., SAFE, S., DE FREITAS, A. S. W., NORSTROM, R. J., WILDISH, D. J. & ZITKO, V. (1972a) Polychlorinated biphenyls: metabolic behaviour of pure isomers in pigeons, rats and brook trout. *Science,* **178**: 312–313.

HUTZINGER, O., SAFE, S. & ZITKO, V. (1971) Polychlorinated biphenyls: Synthesis of some individual chlorobiphenyls. *Bull. environ. Contam. Toxicol.,* **6**: 209–219.

HUTZINGER, O., SAFE, S. & ZITKO, V. (1972b) Photochemical degradation of chlorobiphenyls (PCBs). *Environ. Health Perspect.,* **1**: 15–20.

76

INNAMI, S. *et al.* (1974) PCB toxicity and nutrition II. PCB toxicity and Vitamin A (2). *J. Nutr. Sci-Vitaminol.*, **20**: 363–370.

INTERNATIONAL AGENCY FOR RESEARCH ON CANCER (1974) Polychlorinated biphenyls in IARC monographs on the evaluation of carcinogenic risk of chemicals to man, *Vol. 7*, 261–289.

INTERNATIONAL COUNCIL FOR THE EXPLORATION OF THE SEA (1974) *Report of a Working Group for the international study of the pollution of the North Sea and its effects on living resources and their exploitation.* Charlottenlund, Denmark (Co-operative Research Report No. 39).

ISHI, H. (1972) PCB Pollution in Japan. *Environ. Health Rep. No. 14, Jpn. Publ. Health Assoc.*, pp. 13–28.

ITO, N., NAGASAKI, H., ARAI, M., MAKIURA, S., SUGIHARA, S. & HIRAO, K. (1973) Histopathologic studies on liver tumorigenesis induced in mice by technical polychlorinated biphenyls and its promoting effect on liver tumours induced by benzene hexachloride. *J. nat. Cancer Inst.*, **51**: 1637–1646.

IVERSON, F., VILLENEUVE, D. C., GRANT, D. L. & HATINA, G. V. (1975) Effect of Aroclor 1016 and 1242 on selected enzyme systems in the rat. *Bull. environ. Contam. Toxicol.*, **13**: 456–463.

IWATA, Y., WESTLAKE, W. E. & GUNTHER, F. A. (1973) Varying persistence of polychlorinated biphenyls in six California soils under laboratory conditions. *Bull. environ. Contam. Toxicol.*, **9**: 204–211.

JANSSON, B., JENSEN, S., OLSSON, M., RENBERG, L., SUNDSTRÖM, G. & VAZ, R. (1975) Identification by GC-MS of phenolic metabolites of PCB and p,p'-DDE isolated from Baltic guillemot and seal. *Ambio.*, **4**: 93–97.

JENSEN, S. (1973) (no title) Report to Swedish National Environment Protection Board, Stockholm, 12 October 1973.

JENSEN, S. (1974) *Identification of some organic substances potentially harmful to the environment.* National Swedish Environment Protection Board, University of Stockholm, Kollenberg Laboratory (*Publication SNV-PM 520*).

JENSEN, S. & SUNDSTRÖM, G. (1974) Structures and levels of most chlorobiphenyls in two technical PCB products and in human adipose tissue. *Ambio*, **3**: 70–76.

JENSEN, S. & SUNDSTRÖM, G. (1975) Metabolic hydroxylation of a chlorobiphenyl containing only isolated unsubstituted positions—2,2',4,4',5,5'-hexachlorobiphenyl. *Nature (Lond.)* (in press).

JENSEN, S., JOHNELS, A. G., OLSSEN, M., OTTERLIND, G. (1969) DDT and PCB in marine animals from Swedish waters. *Nature (Lond.)*, **224**: 247–250.

JENSEN, S., JOHNELS, A. G., OLSSON, M. & OTTERLIND, G. (1972b) DDT and PCB in herring and cod from the Baltic, the Kattegat and the Skaggerrak. *Ambio spec. Rep.*, **No. 1**: 71–85.

JENSEN, S., JOHNELS, A. G., OLSSEN, M. & WESTERMARK, T. (1972c) *The avifaune of Sweden as indicators of environmental contamination with mercury and chlorinated hydrocarbons.* In: *Proceedings of the 15th International Ornithology Congress, Leiden*, pp. 455–465.

JENSEN, S., RENBERG, L. & OLSSON, M. (1972a) PCB contamination from boat bottom paint and levels of PCB in plankton outside a polluted area. *Nature (London)*, **240**: 358–360.

JENSEN, S., RENBERG, L. & VAZ, R. (1973) *Problems in quantification of PCB in biological material.* In: *PCB Conference II*. National Swedish Environment Protection Board. Publications: **4E**, pp. 7–13.

JOHANSSON, N., JENSEN, S. & OLSSON, M. (1970) *PCB indications of effects on fish.* In: *PCB Conference*, National Swedish Environment Protection Board, pp. 59–67.

JOHNSTONE, G. J., ECOBICHON, D. J. & HUTZINGER, O. (1974) The influence of pure polychlorinated biphenyl compounds on hepatic function in the rat. *Toxicol. appl. Pharmacol.*, **28**: 66–81.

JONES, D. C. L., DAVIS, W. E., JR, NEWELL, G. W., SASMORE, D. P. & ROSEN, V. J. (1974) Modification of hexachlorophene toxicity by dieldrin and Aroclor 1254. *Toxicology*, **2**: 309–318.

KAISER, K. L. E. & WONG, P. T. S. (1974) Bacterial degradation of polychlorinated biphenyls.

I. Identification of some metabolic products from Aroclor 1242. *Bull. environ. Contam. Toxicol.*, **11**: 291–296.

KARPPANEN, E. & KOLHO, L. (1973) *The concentration of PCB in human blood and adipose tissue in three different research groups.* In: *PCB Conference II.* National Swedish Environment Protection Board Publications: **4E**: pp. 124–127.

KATSUKI, S. (1969) Foreword. *Fukuoka Acta Med.,* **60**: 403–407.

KAWANISHI, S., SANO, S., MIZUTANI, T. & MATSUMOTO, M. (1973) Experimental porphyria induced by polychlorinated biphenyls (in Japanese). *Jpn. J. Hyg.,* **28**: 84.

KAWANISHI, S., SANO, S., MIZUTANI, T. & MATSUMOTO, M. (1974) Experimental studies on toxicity of synthetic tetrachlorobiphenyl isomers (in Japanese). *Jpn. J. Hyg.,* **29**: 81.

KEIL, J. E., PRIESTER, L. E. & SANDIFER, S. H. (1971) Polychlorinated biphenyl (Aroclor 1242): effects of uptake on growth, nucleic acids and chlorophyll of a marine diatom. *Bull. environ. Contam. Toxicol.,* **6**: 156–159.

KEPLINGER, M. L., FANCHER, O. E. & CALANDRA, J. C. (1971) Toxicologic studies with polychlorinated biphenyls. *Toxicol. appl. Pharmacol.,* **19**: 402–403.

KIHLSTROM, J. E., ORBERG, J., LUNDBERG, C., DANIELSSON, P. O. & SYDHOFF, J. (1973) *Effects of PCB on mammalian reproduction.* In: *PCB Conference II.* National Swedish Environment Protection Board Publications **4E**, pp. 109–111.

KIMBROUGH, R. D. (1974) The toxicity of polychlorinated polycyclic compounds and related chemicals. *Crit. Rev. Toxicol.,* **2**: 445–498.

KIMBROUGH, R. D. & LINDER, R. E. (1974) Induction of adenofibrosis and hepatomas of the liver in BALB/cJ mice by polychlorinated biphenyls (Aroclor 1254). *J. nat. Cancer Inst.,* **53**: 547–549.

KIMBROUGH, R. D., LINDER, R. E. & GAINES, T. B. (1972) Morphological changes in livers of rats fed polychlorinated biphenyls. *Arch. environ. Health,* **25**: 354–364.

KIMBROUGH, R. D., LINDER, R. E., BURSE, V. W., JENNINGS, R. W. & GA, C. (1973) Adenofibrosis in the rat liver with persistence of polychlorinated biphenyls in adipose tissue. *Arch. environ. Health,* **27**: 389–395.

KIMBROUGH, R. D., SQUIRE, R. A., LINDER, R. E., STRANDBERG, J. D., MONTALI, R. J. & BURSE, V. W. (1975) Induction of liver tumours in Sherman strain female rats by polychlorinated biphenyl Aroclor 1260. *J. nat. Cancer Inst.,* **55**: 1453–1459.

KIMURA, N. T. & BABA, T. (1973) Neoplastic changes in the rat liver induced by polychlorinated biphenyl. *GANN,* **64**: 105–108.

KITAMURA, M., TSUKAMOTO, T., SUMINO, K., HAYAKAWA, K., SHIBITA, T. & HIRANO, I. (1973) The PCB levels in the blood of workers employed in a condenser factory. *Jpn. J. indust. Health,* **47**: 354–355 (in Japanese).

KOBAYASHI, Y. (1972) Answer Report to the Questionary paper on "Regulation of Residual level in Foods". *Biol. Pollut.,* **4**: 93–116 (in Japanese).

KOEMAN, J. H., TEN NOEVER DE BRAUW & DE VOS, R. H. (1969) Chlorinated biphenyls in fish, mussels and birds from the river Rhine and the Netherlands coastal area. *Nature (Lond),* **221**: 1126–1128.

KOEMAN, J. H., BOTHOF, TH., DE VRIES, R., VAN VELZEN-BLAD, H. & VOS, J. G. (1972a) The impact of persistent pollutants on piscivorous and molluscivorous birds. *TNO-nieuws,* **27**: 561–569.

KOEMAN, J. H., PEETERS, W. H. M., SMIT, C. J., TJIOE, P. S. & DE GOEIJ, J. J. M. (1972b) Persistent chemicals in marine mammals. *TNO-nieuws,* **27**: 570–578.

KOEMAN, J. H., VAN VELZEN-BLAD, H. C. W., DE VRIES, R. & VOS, J. G. (1973) Effects of PCB and DDE in cormorants and evaluation of PCB residues from an experimental study. *J. Reprod. Fertil.,* **19** (Suppl.): 353–364.

KOHANAWA, M., SHOYA, S., OGURA, Y., MORIWAKI, M. & KAWASAKI, M. (1969a) Poisoning due to an oily by-product of rice-bran similar to chick edema disease. I. Occurrence and toxicity test. *Nat. Inst. anim. Health Quart.,* **9**: 213–219.

KOHANAWA, M., SHOYA, S., YONEMURA, T., NISHIMURA, K. & TSUSHIO, Y. (1969b) Poisoning due to an oily by-product of rice-bran similar to chick edema disease. II. Tetrachlorodiphenyl as toxic substance. *Nat. Inst. anim. Health Quart.,* **9**: 220–228.

78

KOLBYE, A. C. JR (1972) Food exposures to polychlorinated biphenyls. *Environ. Health Perspect.*, **1**: 85–88.

KOLLER, L. D. & ZINKL, J. G. (1973) Pathology of polychlorinated biphenyls in rabbits. *Am. J. Pathol.*, **70**: 363–373.

KOMATSU, F. & KIKUCHI, M. (1972) Skin lesions by 3,4,3′,4′-tetrachlorobiphenyl in rabbits. *Fukuoka Acta Med.*, **63**: 384–386 (in Japanese).

KURATSUNE, M. (1972a) PCB pollution. *Kosei no Shihyo*, **19**: 11–18 (in Japanese).

KURATSUNE, M. & MASUDA, Y. (1972b) Polychlorinated biphenyls in non-carbon copypaper. *Environ. Health Perspect.*, **1**: 61–62.

KURATSUNE, M., YOSHIMURA, T. & MATSUZAKA, J. (1972) Epidemiologic study on Yusho, a poisoning caused by ingestion of rice oil contaminated with a commercial brand of polychlorinated biphenyls. *Environ. Health Perspect.*, **1**: 119–128.

KUSUDA, M. (1971) Study on the female sexual function suffering from the chlorobiphenyls poisoning. *Sanka to Fujinka*, **4**: 1063–1072 (in Japanese).

LINCER, J. L. & PEAKALL, D. B. (1970) Metabolic effects of polychlorinated biphenyls in the American kestrel. *Nature (Lond.)*, **228**: 783–784.

LICHTENSTEIN, E. P. (1972) PCBs and interactions with insecticides. *Environ. Health Perspect.*, **1**: 151–153.

LIEB, A. J., BILLS, D. B. & SINNHUBER, R. O. (1974) Accumulation of dietary polychlorinated biphenyls (Aroclor 1254) by rainbow trout (*Salmo gairdneri*). *J. agr. Food Chem.*, **22**: 638–642.

LINDER, R. E., GAINES, T. B. & KIMBROUGH, R. D. (1974) The effect of polychlorinated biphenyls on rat reproduction. *Food cosmet. Toxicol.*, **12**: 63–77.

LITTERST, C. L., FARBER, T. M., BAKER, A. M. & VAN LOON, E. J. (1972) Effect of polychlorinated biphenyls on hepatic microsomal enzymes in the rat. *Toxicol. appl. Pharmacol.*, **23**: 112–122.

MAKIURA, S., AOE, H., SUGIHARA, S., HIRAO, K., ARAI, M. & ITO, N. (1974) Inhibitory effect of polychlorinated biphenyls on liver tumorigenesis in rats treated with 3′-methyl-4-dimethylaminoazobenzene, *N*-2-fluorenylacetamide, and diethylnitrosamine. *J. nat. Cancer Inst.*, **53**: 1253–1257.

MASUDA, Y., KAGAWA, R. & KURATSUNE, M. (1972) Polychlorinated biphenyls in carbonless copying paper. *Nature (Lond.)*, **237**: 41–42.

MASUDA, Y., KAGAWA, R. & KURATSUNE, M. (1974a) Polychlorinated biphenyls in Yusho patients and ordinary persons. *Fukuoka Acta Med.*, **65**: 17–24 (in Japanese).

MASUDA, Y., KAGAWA, R., SHIMAMURA, K., TAKADA, M. & KURATSUNE, M. (1974b) Polychlorinated biphenyls in the blood of Yusho patients and ordinary persons. *Fukuoka Acta Med.*, **65**: 25–27 (in Japanese).

MCKINNEY, J. D. (in press) *Toxicology of selected symmetrical hexachlorobiphenyl isomers: correlating biological effects with chemical structure.* In: *Proceedings of the National Conference on Polychlorinated Biphenyls, Chicago, 19–21 November, 1975.*

MCLAUGHLIN, J. JR., MARLIAC, G. P., VERRETT, M. J., MUTCHLER, M. K. & FITZHUGH, O. G. (1963) The injection of chemicals into the yolk sac of fertile eggs prior to incubation as toxicity test. *Toxicol. appl. Pharmacol.*, **5**: 760–771.

MELVÅS, B. & BRANDT, I. (1973) *The distribution and metabolism of labelled polychlorinated biphenyls in mice and quails.* In: *PCB Conference II.* National Swedish Environment Protection Board Publications: **4E**, pp. 87–90.

MES, J., COFFIN, D. E. & CAMPBELL, D. (1974) Polychlorinated biphenyl and organochlorine pesticide residues in Canadian chicken eggs. *Pestic. Monit. J.*, **8**: 8–11.

MIURA, H., OMORI, S., KATOH, M. (1973) Experimental porphyria in rabbits induced by PCB. *Jpn. J. Hyg.*, **28**: 83 (in Japanese).

MOORE, J. A. (in press) *Toxicity of 2,3,7,8-tetrachlorodibenzofuran: preliminary results. Proceedings of the National Conference on Polychlorinated Biphenyls, Chicago, 19–21 November.*

MOSSER, J. L., FISHER, N. S., TENG, T. & WURSTER, C. F. (1972) Polychlorinated biphenyls: toxicity to certain phytoplankters. *Science*, **175**: 191–192.

MULHERN, B. M., CROMARTIE, E., REICHEL, W. L. & BELISLE, A. A. (1971) Semiquantitative determination of polychlorinated biphenyls in tissue samples by thin layer chromatography. *J. Assoc. Off. Agric. Chem.,* **54**: 548–550.

MURAI, Y. & KUROIWA, Y. (1971) Peripheral neuropathy in chlorobiphenyl poisoning. *Neurol.,* **21**: 1173–1176.

MUSIAL, C. J., HUTZINGER, O., ZITKO, V. & CROCKER, J. (1974) Presence of PCB, DDE and DDT in human milk in the provinces of New Brunswick and Nova Scotia, Canada. *Bull. environ. Contam. Toxicol.,* **12**: 258–267.

NAGAI, J., FURUKAWA, M., YAE, Y. & IKEDA, Y. (1969) Clinicochemical investigation of chlorobiphenyls poisoning. Especially on the serum lipid analysis of the patients. *Fukuoka Acta Med.,* **60**: 475–488 (in Japanese).

NAGAYAMA, J., KURATSUNE, M. & MASUDA, Y. (1976) Determination of chlorinated dibenzofurans in Kanechlors and "Yusho Oil". *Bull. environ. Contam. Toxicol.,* **15**(1): 9–13.

NAGAYAMA, J., MASUDA, Y. & KURATSUNE, M. (1975) Chlorinated dibenzofurans in Kanechlors and rice oils used by patients with Yusho, *Fukuoka Acta Med.,* **66**: 593–599.

NATIONAL SWEDISH ENVIRONMENT PROTECTION BOARD (1973) PCB Conference II. *Publication 1973*: **4E**.

NEBEKER, A. V., PUGLISI, F. A. & DEFOE, D. L. (1974) Effect of polychlorinated biphenyl compounds on survival and reproduction of the fathead minnow and flagfish. *Trans. Am. Fish Soc.,* No. 3, 562–568.

NESTEL, H. & BUDD, J. (1975) Chronic oral exposure of rainbow trout (*Salmo Gairdneri*) to a PCB (Aroclor 1254): pathological effects. *Can. J. comp. Med.,* **39**: 208–215.

NILSSON, B. & RAMEL, C. (1974) Genetic tests on *Drosophila melanogaster* with polychlorinated biphenyls (PCB). *Heriditas,* **77**: 319–322.

NIMMO, D. R., WILSON, P. D., BLACKMAN, R. R. & WILSON, A. J. JR (1971) Polychlorinated biphenyl absorbed from sediments by fiddler crabs and pink shrimp. *Nature (Lond.),* **231**: 50–52.

NISBET, I. C. T. & SAROFIM, A. F. (1972) Rates and routes of transport of PCBs in the environment. *Environ. Health Perspect.* **1**: 21–38.

NISHIMOTO, T., UEDAM, M., TAUL, S. & CHIKAZAWA, K. (1972a) Organochlorine pesticide residues and PCB in breast milk. *Igaku no Ayumi (Proc. Med. Sci.),* **82**: 574–575 (in Japanese).

NISHIMOTO, T., UETA, M., TAUL, S., CHIKAZAURA, K. NISHIUCHI, I. & KONDO, K. (1972b) Deposition of organochlorine pesticide residues and PCB in human body fat. *Igaku no Ayumi (Proc. med. Sci.),* **82**: 515–516.

NISHIZUMI, M. (1970) Light and electron microscope study of chlorobiphenyl poisoning in mouse and monkey liver. *Arch. environ. Health,* **21**: 620–632.

NORÉN, K. & WESTÖÖ, G. (1968) Determination of some chlorinated pesticides in vegetable oils, margarine, butter, milk, eggs, meat and fish by gas chromatography and thin-layer chromatography. *Acta chem. scand.,* **22**: 2289–2293.

ODÉN, S. & BERGGREN, B. (1973) *PCB and DDT in Baltic sediments.* Report Dept. Soil Science, Agricultural College, Uppsala, pp. 1–10.

ODSJÖ, T. (1973) *PCB in some Swedish terrestrial organisms.* In: *PCB Conference II.* National Swedish Environment Protection Board Publications: **4E**, pp. 45–58.

OKUMURA, M. & KATSUKI, S. (1969) Clinical observation on Yusho (chlorobiphenyls poisoning). *Fukuoka Acta Med.,* **60**: 440–446 (in Japanese).

OKUMURA, M., MASUDA, Y. & NAKAMUTA, S. (1974) Correlation between blood PCB and serum triglyceride levels in patients with PCB poisoning. *Fukuoka Acta Med.,* **65**: 84–87 (in Japanese).

OLSSON, M., JENSEN, S. & RENBERG, L. (1973) *PCB in coastal areas of the Baltic. PCB Conference II.* National Swedish Environment Protection Board, Publications: **4E**, pp. 59–68.

ÖRBERG, J. & KIHLSTRÖM, J. E. (1973) Effects of long-term feeding of polychlorinated biphenyls (PCB, Clopehn A60) on the length of the oestrous cycle and on the frequency of implanted ova in the mouse. *Environ. Res.,* **6**: 176–179.

ORGANIZATION FOR ECONOMIC CO-OPERATION AND DEVELOPMENT (1973) *Polychlorinated biphenyls, their use and control.* Environmental Directorate, Paris, OECD.

PANEL ON HAZARDOUS TRACE SUBSTANCES (1972) PCBs—Environmental Impact. *Environ. Res.* **5**: 249–362.

PEAKALL, D. B. LIMIAR, J. L. & BLOOM, S. E. (1972) Embryonic mortality and chromosomal alterations caused by Aroclor 1254 in ring doves. *Environ. Health Perspect.*, **1**: 103–104.

PESENDORFER, VON H., EICHLER, I. & GLOFKE, E. (1973) Informative analyses or organochlorine pesticide and PCB residues in human adipose tissue (from the area of Vienna). *Wiener klinische Wochenschr.*, **85**: 218–222 (summary in English).

PHILLIPS, W. E. J., HATINA, G., VILLENEUVE, D. C. & GRANT, D. L. (1972) Effect of parathion administration in rats following long-term feeding with PCBs. *Environ. physiol. Biochem.*, **2**: 165–169.

PICHIRALLO, J. (1971) PCBs: leaks of toxic substances raises issue of effects, regulations. *Science*, **173**: 899–902.

PLATONOW, N. S. & FUNNELL, H. S. (1971) Anti-androgenic-like effect of polychlorinated biphenyls in cockerels. *Vet. Rec.*, **88**: 109–110.

PLATONOW, N. & CHEN, N. Y. (1973) Transplacental transfer of polychlorinated biphenyls (Aroclor 1254) in a cow. *Vet. Rec.*, **92**: 69–70.

PLATONOW, N. S., FUNNELL, H. S., BULLOCK, D. H., ARNOTT, D. R., SASCHENBRECKER, P. W. & GRIEVE, D. G. (1971) Fate of polychlorinated biphenyls in dairy products processed from the milk of exposed cows. *J. Dairy Sci.*, **54**: 1305–1308.

PLATONOW, N. S., LIPTRAP, R. M. & GEISSINGER, H. D. (1972) The distribution and excretion of polychlorinated biphenyls (Aroclor 1254) and their effect on urinary gonadal steroid levels in the boar. *Bull. environ. Contam. Toxicol.*, **7**: 358–365.

PORTER, M. L., YOUNG, S. J. V. & BURKE, J. A. (1970) A method for the analysis of fish, poultry and animal tissue for chlorinated pesticide residues. *J. Am. Off. Anal. Chem.*, **53**: 1300–1303.

PORTMANN, J. E. (1970) *Monitoring of organochlorine residues in fish from around England and Wales, with special reference to polychlorinated biphenyls.* Report CM 1970/E: 9 International Council for the Exploration of the Sea, Charlottenlund Slot, DK-2920 Charlottenlund, Denmark.

PRESTT, I., JEFFERIES, D. J. & MOORE, N. W. (1970) Polychlorinated biphenyls in wild birds in Britain and their avian toxicity. *Environ. Pollut.*, **1**: 3–26.

PRICE, H. A. & WELCH, R. L. (1972) Occurrence of polychlorinated biphenyls in humans, *Environ. Health Perspect.*, **1**: 73–78.

REHFELD, B. M., BRADLEY, R. L. JR & SUNDE, M. L. (1971) Toxicity studies on polychlorinated biphenyls in the chick. 1. Toxicity and symptoms. *Poult. Sci.*, **50**: 1090–1096.

REINKE, J., UTHE, J. F. & O'BRODOVICH, H. (1973) Determination of polychlorinated biphenyls in the presence of organochlorine pesticides by thin-layer chromatography. *Environ. Lett.*, **4**: 201–210.

REYNOLDS, L. M. (1971) Pesticide residue analysis in the presence of polychlorobiphenyls (PCBs). *Residue Rev.*, **34**: 27–45.

RINGER, R. K., AULERICH, R. J. & ZABIK, M. (1972) Effect of dietary polychlorinated biphenyls on growth and reproduction of mink. *Proc. Amer. chem. Soc.*, 164th A.C.S. Meeting, New York, pp. 149–154.

RISEBROUGH, R. W. & DE LAPPE, B. (1972) Accumulation of polychlorinated biphenyls in ecosystems. *Environ. Health Perspect.*, **1**: 39–45.

RISEBROUGH, R. W., RIECHE, P., PEAKALL, D. B., HERMAN, S. G. & KIRVEN, M. N. (1968) Polychlorinated biphenyls in the global ecosystem. *Nature (Lond.)*, **220**: 1098–1102.

ROACH, J. A. G. & POMERANTZ, I. H. (1974) The finding of chlorinated dibenzofurans in a Japanese polychlorinated biphenyl sample. *Bull. environ. Contam. Toxicol.*, **12**: 338–342.

ROTE, J. W. & MURPHY, P. G. (1971) A method for the quantitation of polychlorinated biphenyl (PCB) isomers. *Bull environ. Contam. Toxicol.*, **6**: 377–384.

SAFE, S. & HUTZINGER, O. (1971) Polychlorinated biphenyls: photolysis of 2,4,6,2′,4′,6′-hexachlorobiphenyl. *Nature (Lond.)*, **232**: 641–642.

SAITO, R., SHIGEMATSU, N. & ISHIMARU, S. (1972) Immunoglobulin levels in serum and sputum of patients with PCB poisoning. *Fukuoka Acta Med.,* **63**: 408–411 (in Japanese).

SANDERS, H. O. & CHANDLER, J. H. (1972) Biological magnification of a polychlorinated biphenyl (Aroclor 1254) from water by aquatic invertebrates. *Bull. environ. Contam. Toxicol.,* **7**: 257–263.

SASCHENBRECKER, P. W., FUNNELL, H. S. & PLATONOW, N. S. (1972) Persistence of polychlorinated biphenyls in the milk of exposed cows. *Vet. Rec.,* **90**: 100–102.

SAVAGE, E. P., TESSARI, J. D., MALBERG, J. W., WHEELER, H. W. & BAGBY, J. R. (1973) A search for polychlorinated biphenyls in human milk in rural Colorado. *Bull. environ. Contam. Toxicol.,* **9**: 222–226.

SCHMIDT, T. T., RISEBROUGH, R. W. & GRESS, F. (1971) Input of polychlorinated biphenyls into California coastal waters from urban sewage outfalls. *Bull. environ. Contam. Toxicol.,* **6**: 235–243.

SCHULTE, E. & ACKER, L. (1974) Gas chromatographic unit Glascapillaran bei Temperaturan bis zu 320°C. *Z. Anal. Chem.,* **268**: 261–267.

SCOTT, M. L., ZIMMERMAN, J. R., MARINSKY, S. & MULLENHOFF, P. A. (1975) Effects of PCBs, DDT and mercury compounds upon egg production, hatchability and shell quality in chickens and Japanese quail. *Poult. Sci.,* **54**: 350–368.

SCHWETZ, B. A., NORRIS, J. M., SPARSCHU, G. L., ROWE, U. K., GEHRING, P. J., EMERSON, J. L. & GERBIG, C. G. (1973) Toxicology of chlorinated dibenzo-*p*-dioxin. *Environ. Health Perspect.,* **5**: 87–99.

SHIGEMATSU, N., NORIMATSU, Y., ISHIBASHI, T., YOSHIDA, M., SUETSUGU, S., KAWATSU, T., IKEDA, T., SAITO, R., ISHIMARU, S., SHIRAKISA, T., KIDO, M., EMORI, K. & TOSHIMITSU, H. (1971) Clinical and experimental studies on respiratory involvement in chlorobiphenyls poisoning. *Fukuoka Acta Med.,* **62**: 150–156 (in Japanese).

SHIGEMATSU, N., ISHIMARU, S., HIROSE, T., IKEDA, T., EMORI, I. & MIYAZAKI, N. (1974) Clinical and experimental studies on respiratory involvement in PCB poisoning. *Fukuoka Acta Med.,* **65**: 88–95 (in Japanese).

SISSONS, D. & WELTI, D. (1971) Structural identification of polychlorinated biphenyls in commercial mixtures by gas–liquid chromatography, nuclear magnetic resonance and mass spectrometry. *J. Chromatogr.,* **60**: 15–32.

SÖDERGREN, A. (1972a) Chlorinated hydrocarbon residues in airborne fallout. *Nature (Lond.),* **236**: 395–397.

SÖDERGREN, A. (1972b) Transport, distribution and degradation of chlorinated hydrocarbon residues in aquatic model ecosystems. *Oikos,* **23**: 30–41.

SÖDERGREN, A. (1973a) Transport, distribution and degradation of DDT and PCB in a south Swedish lake ecosystem. *Vatten,* **2**: 90–108.

SÖDERGREN, A. (1973b) A simplified clean-up technique for organochlorine residues at the microliter level. *Bull. environ. Contam. Toxicol.,* **10**: 116–119.

SÖDERGREN, A. & SVENSSON, Bj. (1973) Uptake and accumulation of DDT and PCB by *Ephemera danica* (Ephemeroptera) in continuous-flow systems. *Bull. environ. Contam. Toxicol.,* **9**: 345–350.

SÖDERGREN, A., SVENSSON, Bj. & ULFSTRAND, S. (1972) DDT and PCB in South Swedish streams. *Environ. Pollut.,* **3**: 25–36.

SOLLY, S. R. B. & SHANKS, V. (1974) Polychlorinated biphenyls and organochlorine pesticides in human fat in New Zealand. *N.Z. J. Sci.,* **17**: 535–544.

SOSA-LUCERO, J. C. & DE LA IGLESIA, F. A. (1973) Distribution of a polychlorinated terphenyl (PCT) (Aroclor 5460) in rat tissues and effect on hepatic microsomal mixed function oxidases. *Bull. environ. Contam. Toxicol.,* **10**: 248–256.

STALLING, D. L. & MAYER, F. L. JR (1972) Toxicities of PCBs to fish and environmental residues. *Environ. Health Perspect.,* **1**: 159–164.

STALLING, D. L., TRINDLE, R. C. & JOHNSON, J. L. (1972) Clean up of pesticides and polychlorobiphenyl residues in fish extracts by gel permeation chromatography. *J. Assoc. Off. Anal. Chem.,* **55**: 32–45.

TAKAMATSU, M., INOUE, Y. & ABE, S. (1974) Diagnostic meaning of the blood PCB. *Fukuoka Acta Med.,* **65**: 28–31 (in Japanese).

82

TAKI, I., HISANAGA, S. & AMAGESE, Y. (1969) Report on Yusho (chlorobiphenyl poisoning). Especially further study of its dermatological findings. *Fukuoka Acta Med.,* **62**: 132–138 (in Japanese).

TAKI, I., KURATSUNE, M., MASUDA, Y. (1973) *Studies on the transmission to the fetus through placenta and the health of mother and baby. Special Research Report on the effects of PCBs on human health such as chronic toxicity for prevention of pollution by PCBs.* Research Co-ordination Bureau, Science and Technology Agency, pp. 87–95 (in Japanese).

TAKIZAWA, Y. & MINAGAWA, K. (1974) Studies on environmental accumulation and bio-accumulation of organochloric compounds. Mainly mentioned PCT. *Studies on the body effect of degradation-registration substances,* pp. 29–50 (in Japanese).

TANAKA, K. & ARAKI, Y. (1974) Inhibitory effect of cholestyramine on the intestinal absorption of PCB. *Fukuoka Acta Med.,* **65**: 53–57.

TANAKA, K. & KOMATSU, F. (1972) Shortening of hexobarbital sleeping time after small doses of PCB in rats. *Fukuoka Acta Med.,* **63**: 360–366 (in Japanese).

TAS, A. C. & DE VOS, R. H. (1971) Characterization of four major components in a technical polychlorinated biphenyl mixture. *Environ. Sci. Technol.,* **5**: 1216–1218.

TATSUKAWA, R. & WATANABE, I. (1972) Air pollution by PCBs. *Shoku No Kagaku,* **8**: 55–63.

THOMAS, G. H. & REYNOLDS, L. M. (1973) Polychlorinated terphenyls in paperboard samples. *Bull. environ. Contam. Toxicol.,* **10**: 37–41.

TREON, J. F., CLEVELAND, F. P., CAPPEL, J. W. & ATCHLEY, R. W. (1956) The toxicity of the vapours of Aroclor 1242 and Aroclor 1254. *Am. Ind. Hyg. Assoc. Quart.,* **17**: 204–213.

TSUKAMOTO, H. ET AL. (1969) The chemical studies on detection of toxic compounds in the rice bran oils used by the patients of Yusho. *Fukuoka Acta Med.,* **60**: 496–512 (in Japanese).

TUCKER, R. K. & CRABTREE, D. G. (1970) *Handbook of toxicity of pesticides to wildlife.* Bureau of Sport, Fisheries and Wildlife Resources Pub. No. 84, Washington, DC, US Dept. of Interior, pp. 130.

TUCKER, E. S., LITSCHGI, W. S. & MEES, W. M. (1975) Migration of polychlorinated bi-phenyls in soil induced by percolating water. *Bull. environ. Contam. Toxicol.,* **13**: 86–93.

URABE, H. (1974) Foreword. *Fukuoka Acta Med.,* **65**: 1–4 (in Japanese).

USDA/USDC/EPA/FDA/USDI/(1972) *Polychlorinated biphenyls and the environment.* Washington DC, Interdepartmental Task Force on PCBs. (Report ITF-PCB-72-1).

USHIO, F., FUKANO, S., NISHIDA, K., KANI, T. & DOGUCHI, M. (1974) Some attempt to estimate the total daily intake of pesticides and PCB residues and trace heavy metals. *Ann. Rep. Tokyo Metr. Res. Lab. P.H.,* **25**: 307–312 (in Japanese).

UTHE, J. F., REINKE, J. & GESSER, H. (1972) Extraction of organochlorine pesticides from water by porous polyurethane coated with selective absorbent. *Environ. Lett.,* **3**: 117–135.

UZAWA, H., ITO, Y., NOTOMI, A. & KATSUKI, S. (1969) Hyperglyceridemia resulting from intake of rice oil contaminated with chlorinated biphenyls. *Fukuoka Acta Med.,* **60**: 449–454 (in Japanese).

UZAWA, H., NOTOMI, A., NAKAMUTA, S. & IKEURA, Y. (1972) Consecutive three year follow up study of serum triglyceride concentrations of 82 subjects with PCB poisoning. *Fukuoka Acta Med.,* **63**: 401–404 (in Japanese).

VAN HOVE HOLDRINET, M. (1975) Preliminary results of an interlaboratory PCB check sample programme. *J. Environ. Qual.* (in press).

VEITH, G. D. (1972) Recent fluctuations of chlorobiphenyls (PCBs) in the Green Bay, Wisconsin, region. *Environ. Health Perspect.,* **1**: 51–54.

VILLENEUVE, D. C., GRANT, D. L., PHILLIPS, W. E. J., CLARK, M. L. & CLEGG, D. J. (1971a) Effects of PCB administration on microsomal enzyme activity in pregnant rabbits. *Bull. environ. Contam. Toxicol.,* **6**: 120–128.

VILLENEUVE, D. C., GRANT, D. L., KHERA, K., CLEGG, D. J., BAER, H. & PHILLIPS, W. E. J. (1971b) The fetotoxicity of a polychlorinated biphenyl mixture (Aroclor 1254) in the rabbit and in the rat. *Environ. Physiol.,* **1**: 67–71.

VILLENEUVE, D. C., GRANT, D. L. & PHILLIPS, W. E. J. (1972) Modification of pentobarbital sleeping times in rats following chronic PCB ingestion. *Bull. environ. Contam. Toxicol.*, 7: 264–269.

VILLENEUVE, D. C., REYNOLDS, L. M., THOMAS, G. H. & PHILLIPS, W. E. J. (1973a) Polychlorinated biphenyls and polychlorinated terphenyls in Canadian food packaging materials. *J. Assoc. Offic. Anal. Chem.*, 56: 999–1001.

VILLENEUVE, D. C., REYNOLDS, L. M. & PHILLIPS, W. E. J. (1973b) Residues of PCBs and PCTs in Canadian and imported European cheeses, Canada-1972. *Pestic. Monit. J.*, 7: 95–96.

VODDEN, H. A. (1973) *Discussion* In: *PCB Conference II.* National Swedish Environment Protection Board, Publications: 4E, p. 118.

VOS, J. G. (1972) Toxicology of PCBs for mammals and for birds. *Env. Health Perspect.*, 1: 105–117.

VOS, J. G. & BEEMS, R. B. (1971) Dermal toxicity studies of technical polychlorinated biphenyls and fractions thereof in rabbits. *Toxicol. appl. Pharmacol.*, 19: 617–633.

VOS, J. G. & DE ROIJ, Th. (1972) Immunosuppressive activity of a polychlorinated biphenyl preparation on the humoral immune response in guinea pigs. *Toxicol. appl. Pharmacol.*, 21: 549–555.

VOS, J. G. & KOEMAN, J. H. (1970) Comparative toxicologic study with polychlorinated biphenyls in chickens with special reference to porphyria, edema formation, liver necrosis and tissue residues. *Toxicol. appl. Pharmacol.*, 17: 656–668.

VOS, J. G. & NOTENBOOM-RAM, E. (1972) Comparative toxicity study of 2,4,5,2′,4′,5′-hexachlorobiphenyl and a polychlorinated biphenyl mixture in rabbits. *Toxicol. appl. Pharmacol.*, 23: 563–578.

VOS, J. G. & VAN DRIEL-GROOTENHUIS, L. (1972) PCB-induced suppression of the humoral and cell-mediated immunity in guinea pigs. *Sci. Total Environ.*, 1: 289–302.

VOS, J. G., KOEMAN, J. H., VAN DER MAAS, H. L,, TEN NOEVER DE BRAUW, M. G. & DE VOS, R. E. (1970) Identification and toxicological evaluation of chlorinated dibensofuran and chlorinated naphthalene in two commercial polychlorinated biphenyls. *Fd. cosmet. Toxicol.*, 8: 625–633.

VOS, J. G., STRIK, J. J. T. W. A., VAN HOLSTEYN, C. M. W. & PENNINGS, J. H. (1971) Polychlorinated biphenyls as inducers of hepatic porphyria in Japanese quail, with special reference to δ-aminolevulinic acid synthetase activity, fluorescence and residues in the liver. *Toxicol. appl. Pharmacol.*, 20: 232–240.

WEBB, R. G. & McCALL, A. C. (1972) Identification of polychlorinated biphenyl isomers in aroclors. *J. Am. Off. Anal. Chem.*, 55: 746–752.

WESTÖÖ, G. & NORÉN, K. (1970a) Levels of organochlorine pesticides and polychlorinated biphenyls in fish caught in Swedish water areas or kept for sale in Sweden, 1967–1970. *Var Föda*, 3: 93–146 (summary in English).

WESTÖÖ, G. & NORÉN, K. (1970b) Determination of organochlorine pesticides and polychlorinated biphenyls in animal foods. *Acta Chem. Scand.*, 24: 1639–1644.

WESTÖÖ, G. & NORÉN, K. (1972) Levels of organochlorine pesticides and polychlorinated biphenyls in Swedish human milk. *Var Föda*, 24: 41–54 (summary in English).

WESTÖÖ, G., NORÉN, K. & ANDERSSON, M. (1971) Levels of organochlorine pesticides and polychlorinated biphenyls in some cereal products. *Var Föda*, 10: 341–360 (summary in English).

WHO WORKING GROUP (1973) *The hazzards to health and ecological effects of persistent substances in the environment—polychlorinated biphenyls.* Report of a Working Group convened by the World Health Organization, Regional Office for Europe, EURO, 3109(2).

WILDISH, D. J. (1970) The toxicity of polychlorinated biphenyls (PCB) in sea water to *Grammarus oceanicus. Bull. environ. Contam. Toxicol.*, 5: 202–204.

WILLIAMS, R. & HOLDEN, A. V. (1973) Organochlorine residues from plankton. *Mar. Pollut. Bull.*, 4, 109–111.

WILLIS, D. E. & ADDISON, R. F. (1972) Identification and estimation of the major components of a commercial polychlorinated biphenyl mixture, *Aroclor 1221. J. Fish. Res. Board Can.*, **29**(5): 592–595.

WONG, P. T. S. & KAISER, K. L. E. (1975) Bacterial degradation of polychlorinated biphenyls. II. Rate studies. *Bull. environ. Contam. Toxicol.,* **13**: 249–256.

YAGAMUCHI, A., YOSHIMURA, T. & KURATSUNE, M. (1971) A survey on pregnant women having consumed rice oil contaminated with chlorobiphenyls and their babies. *Fukuoka Acta Med.,* **62**: 112–117 (in Japanese).

YAMAMOTO, H. & YOSHIMURA, H. (1973) Metabolic studies on polychlorinated biphenyls. III. Complete structure and acute toxicity of the metabolites of 2,4,3′,4′-tetrachlorobiphenyl. *Chem. pharm. Bull.,* **21** (10): 2237–2242 (in English).

YOBS, A. R. (1972) Levels of polychlorinated biphenyls in adipose tissue of the general population of the nation. *Environ. Health Perspect.,* **1**: 79–81.

YOSHIMURA, T. (1971) Epidemiological analysis of "Yusho" patients with special reﬁrence to sex, age, clinical grades and oil consumption. *Fukuoka Acta Med.,* **62**: 109–116 (in Japanese).

YOSHIMURA, H. & YAMAMOTO, H. (1973) Metabolic studies on polychlorinated biphenyls. I. Metabolic fate of 3,4,3′,4′-tetrachlorobiphenyl in rats. *Chem. pharm. Bull.,* **21**: 1168–1169 (in English).

YOSHIMURA, H. & YAMAMOTO, H. (1974) Metabolic studies on polychlorinated biphenyls. IV. Biotransformation of 3,4,3′,4′-tetrachlorobiphenyl, one of the major components of Kanechlor-400. *Fukuoka Acta Med.,* **65**: 5–11 (in Japanese).

YOSHIMURA, H. & YAMAMOTO, H. (1975) A novel route of excretion of 2,4,3′,4′-tetrachlorobiphenyl in rats. *Bull. environ. Contam. Toxicol.,* **13**: 681–687.

YOSHIMURA, H., YAMAMOTO, H., NAGAI, J., YAE, Y., UZAWA, H., ITO, Y., NOTOMI, A., MIMAKAMI, S., ITO, A., KATO, K. & TSUJI, H. (1971) Studies on the tissue distribution and the urinary and faecal excretion of ^{3}H-Kanechlor (chlorobiphenyls) in rats. *Fukuoka Acta Med.,* **62**: 12–19 (in Japanese).

YOSHIMURA, H., YAMAMOTO, H. & SAEKI, S. (1973) Metabolic studies on polychlorinated biphenyls. II. Metabolic fate of 2,4,3′4′-tetrachlorobiphenyl in rats. *Chem. pharm. Bull.,* **21**: 2231–2236 (in English).

YOSHIMURA, H., YAMAMOTO, H. & KINOSHITA, H. (1974) Metabolic studies on polychlorinated biphenyls. V. Biliary excretion of 5-hydroxy-2,4,3′,4′,-tetrachlorobiphenyl, a major metabolite of 2,4,3′,4′-tetrachlorobiphenyl. *Fukuoka Acta Med.,* **65**: 12–16 (in Japanese).

ZIMMERLI, B. & MAREK, B. (1973) Die Belastung der Schweizerischen Bevölkerung mit Pestiziden. *Mitt. Lebensm. Unters. Hyg.,* **64**: 459–479.

ZITKO, V. (1970) Polychlorinated biphenyls (PCB) solubilized in water by nonionic surfactants for studies of toxicity to aquatic animals. *Bull. environ. Contam. Toxicol.,* **5**: 279–285.

ZITKO, V. (1971) Polychlorinated biphenyls and organochlorine pesticides in some freshwater and marine fishes. *Bull. environ. Contam. Toxicol.,* **6**: 464–470.

ZITKO, V., HUTZINGER, O. & SAFE, S. (1971) Retention times and electron-capture detector responses of some individual chlorobiphenyls. *Bull. environ. Contam. Toxicol.,* **6**: 160–163.

ZITKO, V., HUTZINGER, O., JAMIESON, W. D. & CHOI, P. M. K. (1972a) Polychlorinated terphenyls in the environment. *Bull. environ. Contam. Toxicol.,* **7**: 200–201.

ZITKO, V., HUTZINGER, O. & CHOI, P. M. K. (1972b) Contamination of the Bay of Fundy—Gulf of Maine area with polychlorinated biphenyls, polychlorinated terphenyls, chlorinated dibenzodioxins and dibenzofurans. *Environ. Health Perspect.,* **1**: 47–50.

ZITKO, V., CHOI, P. M. K., WILDISH, D. J., MONAGHAN, C. F. & LISTER, N. A. (1974) Distribution of PCBs and *p,p′*-DDE residues in Atlantic herring and yellow perch in eastern Canada, 1972. *Post. Mon. J.,* **8**: 105–109.

WORLD HEALTH ORGANIZATION PUBLICATIONS

SUBSCRIPTIONS AND PRICES 1977

Global Subscription

The global subscription covers all WHO publications, i.e., the combined subscription IV and, in addition, the Monograph Series and non-serial publications, including the books, but not the slides, of the International Histological Classification of Tumour series and not the publications of the International Agency for Research on Cancer.   US $440.00   Sw. fr. 1,100.

Combined Subscriptions

Special prices are offered for combined subscriptions to certain publications as follows:

Subscription

I *Bulletin, Chronicle, Technical Report Series* and *Public Health Papers*   US $96.00   Sw. fr.   240.—

II *World Health Statistics Report* and *World Health Statistics Annual*   US $104.00   Sw. fr.   260.—

III *World Health Statistics Report, World Health Statistics Annual* and *Weekly Epidemiological Record*   US $140.00   Sw. fr.   350.—

IV *Bulletin, Chronicle, Technical Report Series, Public Health Papers, WHO Offset Publications, Official Records, International Digest of Health Legislation, World Health Statistics Report, World Health Statistics Annual, Weekly Epidemiological Record, WHO Regional Publications* and *World Health*   US $340.00   Sw. fr.   850.—

The World Health Organization will be pleased to submit a quotation for any other type of combined subscription desired.

Individual Subscriptions

Bulletin, vol. 55 (one volume only—six numbers)	US $36.00	Sw. fr. 90.—
Chronicle, vol. 31 (12 numbers)	US $18.00	Sw. fr. 45.—
International Digest of Health Legislation, vol. 28 (4 numbers)	US $34.00	Sw. fr. 85.—
Technical Report Series	US $40.00	Sw. fr. 100.—
Official Records	US $40.00	Sw. fr. 100.—
World Health Statistics Report, vol. 30	US $40.00	Sw. fr. 100.—
Weekly Epidemiological Record, 52nd year (52 numbers)	US $44.00	Sw. fr. 110.—
Vaccination Certificate Requirements for International Travel	US $7.20	Sw. fr. 18.—
WHO Regional Publications	US $20.00	Sw. fr. 50.—
World Health, vol. 30	US $10.00	Sw. fr. 25.—

International Agency for Research on Cancer Subscription

Annual Report, IARC Monographs on the evaluation of Carcinogenic Risk of Chemicals to Man, and *IARC Scientific Publications*   US $120.00   Sw. fr.   300.—

Subscriptions can be obtained from WHO sales agents for the calendar year only (January to December).   Prices are subject to change without notice.

2961—1

5-07

*
*   *

Specimen numbers of periodicals and a catalogue will be sent free of charge on request.